Mad Scientist Muscle

Build Monster Mass With Science-Based Training

By Nick Nilsson

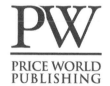

PRICE WORLD
PUBLISHING

Mad Scientist Muscle: Build Monster Mass With Science-Based Training

First Edition 2012

ISBN: 9781932549799

eISBN: 9781936910168

Library of Congress Control Number: 2011916300

Prior to beginning any exercise program, you must consult with your physician. You must also consult your physician before increasing the intensity of your training.

Any application of the recommended material in this book is at the sole risk of the reader, and at the reader's discretion. Responsibility of any injuries or other negative effects resulting from the application of any of the information provided within this book is expressly disclaimed.

Published by Price World Publishing

1300 W. Belmont Ave. Suite #20g

Chicago, IL 60657

For information about discounts for bulk purchases, please contact info@priceworldpublishing.com.

Printing by Sheridan Books

Printed in the United States of America

10 9 8 7 6 5 4 3 2 1

Table of Contents

Introduction

The Program

Exercise

The Core Combo

Nutrition

Appendix

References

Suggested Reading

**This program is all about building muscle and building it FAST
with unique, targeted, science-based approaches...
...and yes, a little bit of insanity here and there :)**

You see, in my 20+ years in the gym, I've read a LOT of books and studies on muscle, fat-loss and exercise and yes, even many of those "evil" muscle magazines.

I've also spent literally <u>THOUSANDS</u> of hours creating and innovating new exercises and training techniques with some pretty incredible results (that's where my nickname as the "Mad Scientist of Exercise" came about).

The two pictures below are of me...the purpose of which is to show you that **I practice what I preach**. I love to train for MASS and I love training with heavy weight.

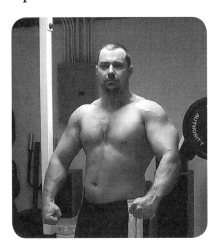 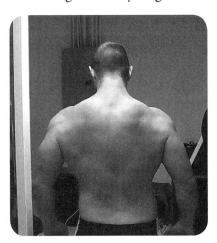

So Enough About Me...What Is Mad Scientist Muscle?

Glad you asked! Let's get right into it...

First, in this mass-building program, you're going to be strategically manipulating the types of training you're doing along with the volume, the frequency and the intensity in order to literally FORCE your body to grow.

Second, you're also going to be using a number of very targeted, very specialized training techniques designed to physically

CHANGE the underlying structure of your body to help better support muscle growth. I'll explain...

"Mad Scientist" Principle #1
Planned Overtraining and Rebound

The core program structuring principle you'll be putting to work is known by many names..."**Accumulation and Intensification**" **and "Dual Factor Theory"** are two of the most common.

As far as this base concept goes, I definitely won't pretend that I created it... it's been around for a <u>LONG</u> time in various forms and has been used and talked about by many top coaches and trainers such as Charles Poliquin, Charlie Francis, and many Eastern Bloc coaches.

There is a tremendous amount of research on the subject and I could give you a HUGELY detailed physiological explanation of how it all works but I have a feeling you'd rather just know how it's going to build muscle on you :)

So here goes...

Basically, for a period of a few weeks, you will increase your workload by increasing training volume (number of sets for each body part) and decreasing rest periods between sets until you get to the point at or near overtraining. This is "**accumulation**" as you're accumulating workload and fatigue on the body and demanding more of it than that is currently able to recover fully from.

When you REACH that point, you then back off and dramatically reduce the training volume, doing fewer sets, while also increasing rest periods between sets. This is the "**intensification**" part of things and it's where the REAL growth happens.

Here's what it looks like graphical form...the white area in the in middle is the "optimal" zone for muscle growth. As you can see, you're spending a LOT of time there with this program!

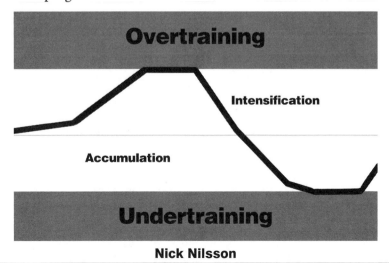

Overtraining

Intensification

Accumulation

Undertraining

Nick Nilsson

When you begin the program, you gradually accumulate workload and training volume, moving more and more towards overtraining. This training "on the edge" is where the REAL results are - you won't get anywhere if you stay too far away from it.

At the end of the "accumulation" phase, you've hit Overtraining. THAT is when we back off and reduce the training volume, increase rest periods and start using heavier weights. This "intensification" will gradually move you towards "undertraining" as your body adapts to the reduced workload.

This is followed by a deloading phase where you pull WAY back on your training and allow your body to more fully recover before you start ramping back up in the next training cycle.

Think of a car going up a hill with the gas pedal down. As you come to the top, you've got the pedal floored but you're not going very fast...you're overtraining the engine, to borrow a term you might be familiar with.

Now you go over the top and start heading down the other side. If you keep that pedal floored, you're going to start going

VERY fast! Your body/engine is no longer overtrained by the steep grade but it's still pushing just as hard.

THAT is the power of this type of training. You're going to systematically push your body's gas pedal to the point where you have it floored and aren't really going anywhere, then you're going to pull back and let it ROAR forward. The results you get from this type of overtraining and rebounding can be <u>HUGE</u> and THAT is what each of these three programs will do for you.

Now here's an eye-opener for you...

With "normal" training programs that don't take your body's response to workload into account, you can get into either of two outcomes, neither of which is desirable.

In the graph below, you'll see two lines...the top graph line is "Too Much Volume/Intensity." The bottom graph line is "Not Enough Volume/Intensity." Both hypothetical training programs spend time in the optimal training zone and both will get you results for awhile...

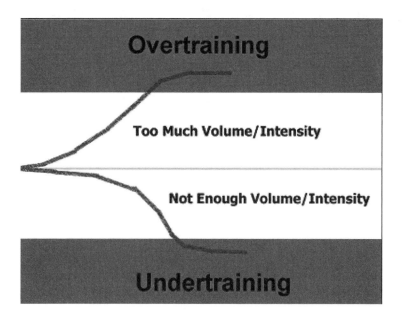

In the top line, the problem happens when the program DOESN'T PULL BACK. You hit overtraining and your body stops getting results. The usual response? Add even MORE volume and/or intensity. This can result in chronic overtraining and hitting a MAJOR plateau in your training. The only cure is backing off.

In the bottom line, the problem happens when your body adapts and you DON'T INCREASE volume or intensity...i.e. you keep doing what you're doing. This is chronic UNDER-training and it'll put a stop to your results, too.

"Accumulation and Intensification" is the Cure...

So what I've done is taken this core framework of "**planned overtraining and rebound**" and created three programs using THE most effective muscle-and-strength-building techniques and training session structures I've read about or come up with myself in my 20+ "mad scientist" years in the gym.

Each program is packed with very powerful training techniques designed to build MASSIVE muscle all structured on this type of volume/intensity-driven format. And each program offers a varying degree of difficulty.

All of these programs attack muscle growth on a SYSTEMIC level...you're going to be using the adaptive power of your entire body as a system rather than trying to grow body parts in isolation.

"Mad Scientist" Principle #2

Training to Change Your Physiology to Better Support Muscle Growth

When it comes right down it, there are real physiological reasons why some people don't gain muscle quickly and some do. There are some factors you can't do anything about (e.g. genetics, predominant muscle-fibers types, and basic hormonal make-up) but there are MANY factors you can focus on in your training that can actually change your base physiology to make it more favorable to muscle growth.

I like to compare it to building a house...

You're going to be able to build a bigger, better house (i.e. muscle mass) when the walls and beams are thicker and stronger (bones and connective tissue), the plumbing is better (your circulatory system) and your electrical system is more efficient (your nervous system).

In each of the three program cycles, I've included specific Structural Training that's going to address these base physiological factors and change them for the better. It's going to make it easier for you to build muscle, no matter what your level of ability to gain muscle mass is currently at!

I'll go into a lot more detail on exactly how this is done and what type of training you'll be doing in the Structural Training chapter of the program.

Now, in addition to the base training structure and the structural training, I've also included a special nutritional tweak to help minimize body fat gain while setting up even BETTER muscle gains every week. It's an optional tweak but I've experienced phenomenal results with it. You may have used it before but probably not in a muscle-building program!

Bottom line, you put these two "Mad Scientist" principles together and you will get EXPLOSIVE results. This stuff flat-out WORKS.

Your body is naturally programmed to respond to cyclical training like this and it simply has no choice but to get bigger!

Nick Nilsson

The "Mad Scientist " of the Fitness World

How to Use This Book

S tart by reading through the entire book before beginning the workouts. The first section, **The Programs**, includes an overview of how the programs work, how all the pieces fit together and etc...

The other sections of the book (**Exercises** and **Nutrition**) provide more detailed information about the different exercise and nutritional aspects of the program.

Be sure to read through all the sections before you start the program so you will understand the aims of the program and how it works. Knowing how it works will help you get the best results!

The Program

In this book I've included **THREE 8-week** training programs (that's six months of training!) for you to use and experiment with. These will keep you getting great results and keep your training FUN for a LONG time!

You can do these training cycles in ANY order, so if any one cycle appeals to you more, you're free to start with that. Each one can stand alone on its own.

Cycle 1 - Time/Volume Training

Week 1 - Structural

Week 2 - Volume - Time/Volume 1

Week 3 - Volume - Time/Volume 2

Week 4 - Volume - Time/Volume 3

Week 5 - Structural

Week 6 - Intensity - Low-Rep Strength Training 1

Week 7 - Intensity - Low-Rep Strength Training 2

Week 8 - OFF/Deload/Fun/Strength Test

View the Program Outline and Workouts in the Appendix on page TC

Cycle 2 - Cluster Training

Week 1 - Structural

Week 2 - Volume - Cluster Training 1

Week 3 - Volume - Cluster Training 2

Week 4 - Volume - Cluster Training 3

Week 5 - Structural

Week 6 - Intensity - Single Rep Cluster Training 1

Week 7 - Intensity - Single Rep Cluster Training 2

Week 8 - OFF/Deload/Fun/Strength Test

View the Program Outline and Workouts in the Appendix on page TC

Cycle 3 - Rest-Pause Training

Week 1 - Structural

Week 2 - Volume - Rest-Pause Training 1

Week 3 - Volume - Rest-Pause Training 2

Week 4 - Volume - Rest-Pause Training 3

Week 5 - Structural

Week 6 - Intensity - Triple Add Sets 1

Week 7 - Intensity - Triple Add Sets 2

Week 8 - OFF/Deload/Fun/Strength Test

View the Program Outline and Workouts in the Appendix on page TC

Take Pictures!

I highly recommend taking **"Before & After"** pictures and just before you start and just after you finish the program.

The differences in your body will really amaze you. It's extremely motivating to be able to see the rapid improvements you've made!

How and Why It Works

This section will tell exactly why it all works when combined and timed the way it is. This will be a point-by-point look at how each aspect of the program fits in with the others to get the best results. It's like watching a "Making Of" special on your favorite movie! This will allow you to understand the program and make changes to it for yourself as you get more experienced with it. What works well for one person may work like crazy for the next!

Through each phase of the program, you'll be able to exercise the "Low-Carb Option" on the weekends, if you wish. This means eating low-carb for two days (on non-training days) to help minimize fat gain and to set up a bigger weight gain rebound during the week. I will explain all of the benefits of this technique of this in the **Nutrition** section of the book but remember: it is optional!

The Nuts and Bolts of Structural Training:

In the Structural Training phase of the program, we're not specifically looking to gain muscle...we're looking to build and enhance the physiological BASE upon which to build muscle.

One of the main reasons people are hardgainers or have problem body parts is that the physiology of their body isn't developed well enough to support extra muscle mass. Muscle is metabolically costly...our job here is to make it EASIER for your body to build and hold onto that muscle by greasing the wheels and reducing the metabolic cost of having that muscle...make it more efficient to build and maintain.

The first two days of this section utilize higher rep ranges and faster movements to accomplish two things...increase the microcirculation (i.e. capillarization) going to your muscles and "wake up" the nervous system.

By increasing the microcirculation, we'll improve the ability of your body to deliver oxygen and nutrients and remove waste products. By using speed and explosive-based movements, we'll be improving nervous system function by teaching your body to activate more motor units during exercises, which increases strength.

The two days also include stretch-focused exercises immediately after each high-rep set. When the muscle is filled with blood, the stretch-focused exercise will help stretch the fascia (the connective-tissue sheath surrounding the muscle), giving the muscles more room to grow.

The second two training days are dedicated to heavier, low-rep partial training. The idea here is also twofold...first, to load the connective tissue and muscles with extremely heavy weight and second, to again target the nervous system to get accustomed to moving heavier loads than normal.

This Structural Training is repeated twice in each cycle of the program and is the same in all three cycles.

The Nuts and Bolts of Volume Training:

This can also be described as the "Accumulation" phase of the program where you will be accumulating training volume and gradually overloading the body in order to force it to adapt to ever-increasing workloads.

The analogy I like to use is a car going up a steep hill...you have it floored as you come to the top and you're still going slow, but when you come over the top and start going down the other side, you pick up speed FAST!

THAT is the basis of what we're trying to accomplish with this type of training and it's accomplished in different ways in each unique cycle of the program.

In Time/Volume Training, you'll be increasing your training density each session, attempting to do more and more reps within a specific timeframe. When you hit the goal for workload, you increase the weight the next time, so over the course of three weeks, you will gradually be increasing the overall workload on your muscles.

In Cluster Training, we'll be gradually increasing the number of Cluster sets you're doing while decreasing rest periods within the sets. This is another way of increasing training density and workload.

With Rest-Pause Training, we're going to gradually increase the number of Rest-Pause sets done along with forcing incremental increases in resistance used. The in-set rest periods will remain the same.

This Volume-based training is going to push you towards the point of overtraining and that's a GOOD thing!

The Nuts and Bolts of Intensity Training:

This is the "Intensification" phase of the program (where you're in the car and now you're coming down the other side of the hill!). The high volume work you put in on the previous phase is now going to pay off as your body is still cranking, trying to recover from the uphill workload of the previous phase.

We'll take a lower-volume, higher-intensity approach to training here; doing fewer sets, using more weight and really building some serious strength. Rest periods will be relatively long compared to the first phase...the goal is performance. We won't be increasing workload or decreasing rest periods...just focusing on adding resistance when possible.

In the first cycle, this will be done with Low Rep Strength Training. This is a simple, straightforward approach that utilizes a scheme of 5-3-1 reps...no intensity techniques, just low-rep strength training with heavy weight.

In the second cycle, you'll use Single Rep Cluster Training, which has you doing 1 rep mini-sets of about 90% of your max. You repeat these mini-sets with minimal rest for a total of 8 to 10 reps. This allows you to get more reps with near-maximal weight. You will also be utilizing Bottom Start Single Rep Cluster Training to remove elastic tension from the movements and force the muscles to do ALL the work.

In the third cycle, you'll be doing Triple Add Sets. This utilizes more of an "intensity technique" type of style with a very specific goal...to target ALL the major muscle fiber types in one set. It's a very intense technique so you won't be doing very many of them but they strongly hit every single fiber type you've got all at once.

These Intensification phases will help you achieve fast increases in strength and muscle mass as your body gets more and more efficient and "comes down" from the overloading of the Volume/Accumulation phases.

The Nuts and Bolts of Deload/Fun/Strength Test Training:

Once you've completed the Intensity phase, it's time to give your body a bit of a break. It's important to give your body that time off from training to rebuild and recover.

I've given you a couple of options in this phase of the program. You'll be taking 4 days off, coming off the Intensity phase, before you train again. On one of the days, you'll have the option to train, if you feel up to it. On that day, you'll be doing fun and unique exercises that utilize unique movement patterns and address weak points in some of your lifts.

This day is optional - if you feel your nervous system and overall recovery needs it, then you can take the day off completely.

The fifth day of the cycle is a "max out" day where we'll be testing your strength on some of the big lifts to gauge your progress. Max-out days are only done once every two months - doing them more frequently just isn't that useful as a true 1 Rep Max is very demanding on the body. After 2 months of training, you will see some big changes in your numbers!

The Sum of All Parts:

The real power of this program lies in the overall systemic effect on the body, not necessarily in the individual training sessions. We set the stage for increased muscle growth by purposefully adapting the body's physiology to better support muscle growth. Then we increase the workload on the body to force it towards overtraining. Then we back off on workload and focus on increasing strength.

This wavelike approach yields tremendous short-term results and is the ONLY practical way to achieve sustained long-term results as well. You're working WITH your body's natural adaptation reaction to training, not against it.

It's a powerful structure that consistently yields excellent results - each of the three cycles of the program work this type of pattern in a different way, keeping things interesting and unique for the long-term.

Excercise

Exercise is the cornerstone of this program and where my REAL "Mad Scientist" stuff comes out! You may be familiar with a few of these training techniques...and if so, you may see them being used in ways you've never seen before.

Read through each section and be sure you understand what to do and why. The more you know and understand, the better you will be able to adjust the training for your own specific body and the more effective this training program will be.

Using Overtraining for GOOD Not Evil...	Learn how you can take what is normally considered bad for you (overtraining) and make it into something that will help you get continuous, spectacular results!
Structural Training	This is the base of the program...the techniques that will build the circulation and structure of your body to help support increased muscle mass.
Cluster Training	This training method is geared towards building and keeping muscle while burning fat. When used in combination with the programs and nutrition in this book, you may even make better muscle gains than in your regular mass training.
Time/Volume Training	This style of training is all about short sets, managed rest and high volume. It's an ideal way to achieve muscle mass gains even with bodyweight exercises you can do a LOT of reps with.
Rest-Pause Training	This is a powerful training technique that pushes your muscles beyond chemical failure.
Triple Add Sets	This technique uses 3 different rep and weight ranges to target every single fiber type in your muscles all in one shot.

Low Rep Strength Training	Develop your maximal strength with very low-rep training.
Deload/Fun/ Strength Test	You need to back off your training in order to keep your body recovering and building. This is built-in and scripted.
Aerobic Interval Training	Learn exactly how to perform Aerobic Interval Training that is an optional part of this program.
The Core Combo	The Core Combo has three main components designed to improve your abdominal and lower back strength and definition. It also includes exercises for the Rotator Cuff to keep your shoulders strong and healthy.
How to Max Out	Learn the best way to work up to your maximum lifts without tiring yourself out by warming up TOO much. It's a fine line - learn how to do it right.

Using Overtraining For
FASTER Results

**We've always been told that it's bad to overtrain. Guess what?
Overtraining on purpose is where the REAL results are.**

O vertraining is NOT evil. Overtraining can be exactly what you need to achieve continuous and rapid results in your training. We will be applying the concept of strategically-designed, temporary overtraining to the Mad Scientist Muscle program cycles to ensure you make continuous gains.

But first, what is overtraining? Overtraining is, most simply, training too much. Your body is unable to recover from the volume or frequency of training and begins to break down. You not only lose motivation to train, you become more susceptible to injury and illness, and you may even start to go backwards in your training, getting smaller and weaker on almost a daily basis.

So how can overtraining possibly be good for you? I'll tell you.

It all begins with the incredible adaptive power of your body. As you become more advanced in weight training, you will generally notice that you cannot make consistent gains for a long period of time on one training system. Your body quickly adapts to whatever training system you're using and hits a plateau. To get around this, it's usually recommended that you change your program every three to six weeks.

The question now is how to use this adaptive ability to your advantage.

It's really quite simple. You gradually build up to a state of temporary overtraining, then, when you're overtrained and your adaptive processes are working to their fullest capacity for recovery, you back off. This results in what is called overcompensation.

Imagine you're driving a car and climbing a hill with the gas pedal to the floor. You're giving it everything you've got but you're still going up slowly. This is similar to overtraining. When you reach the top, the going gets a lot easier. If you keep the gas pedal on the floor when you go over the top and head down, you're going to go a lot faster very quickly.

This is overcompensation and this is where the results are.

In a normal program, you work a body part, it becomes temporarily weaker, then becomes stronger as it overcompensates so you can lift more next time. What a normal program does on a small, local basis, this targeted overtraining does on a full body, systemic basis.

Sound good? We're not done. Now we're going to harness the power of overtraining by using what I call **"Controlled Overtraining."** This idea goes by many other names but the core concept remains the same...

Accumulation:

As you go through the first phase of each cycle, you'll notice that the number of sets/workload you're doing increases. By starting at a lower volume and gradually building up the training volume, you are forcing your body to adapt. When you get to the final phase before backing off, you'll be maxing out on training volume and your metabolism will be cranking strongly to keep up. At this point, you will start to become somewhat overtrained.

This ramping up phase is known as "Accumulation." You're accumulating training volume, forcing your body to perform more and work more.

Intensification:

This is where we back off.

You will change both your training style and your nutrition. You will target your training to strength-building, decreasing the number of sets and reps and increasing the rest periods.

This is called "Intensification" because the intensity of the training is increasing (intensity, in technical terms, means how close to your 1 rep max you're training at - the closer you are to that maximum, the higher the intensity of your training - it has nothing to do with how hard you grimace or how loud you scream while training).

This backing-off allows you to recover from the overtraining and take advantage of the overcompensation that occurs when the body is still working at dealing with the hard work and then you cut the hard work. Though it may feel like you're hardly doing anything at all, you should see some great results both in strength and muscle mass increases.

The back-off period is crucial for the body to recuperate and regenerate, especially if you are planning to move to the next cycle of the program. This period will help you to avoid chronic overtraining, which will send your results plummeting.

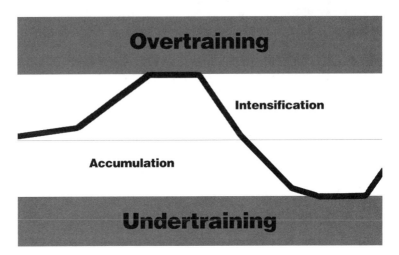

Keeping up this cycling of volume and intensity is a strategy that gives consistent results in fat loss, muscle gain and strength over long periods of time. **It will allow you to get big, lean and strong all at the same time.**

As you can see, overtraining is not always the horrible thing it's often made out to be. Training on the edge is where the real results are. Those who shy away from it will never make as good of progress as those who embrace it.

How to Know When to Pull Back and Should You Adjust the Program?

While it is true that the best program is one that's perfectly tailored to your recovery ability, I highly recommend going through the program as-is the first time you use it.

The accumulation phase starts off relatively easy. You shouldn't have any problem completing the sets. As it progresses, you may find you hit the overtraining wall sooner than others.

In this case, if you feel that happening, I recommend keeping the sets to the same as you did the previous week while still reducing the rest periods between sets. This will still give you the overtraining stimulus we're looking for while reducing the load on the body somewhat to allow it to continue.

The intensification phases are low volume and should be fine for the majority of people as they're designed to basically detrain you in terms of volume, allowing for greater recovery.

Structural Training

Structural Training is going to build your muscle "base"...the plumbing, the electric system and the structure that's going to help you make the best use of the actual "building" training you'll be doing during the other phases of the program.

This week of training is not about building muscle directly...it's about SETTING THE STAGE for improved rate of muscle building in the rest of the program. It's important not to skip this week or slack off on it. This is the training that's going to prepare your body for maximum growth.

DAY 1

The first training day is going to entail moderate weight with fairly high reps (20+ reps per set). You'll be doing these with FAST speed. This will help fire up the nervous system along with helping you squeeze out more reps.

This will also force a LOT of blood into the muscles, helping increase microcirculation to the muscles as well as overall vascularity (which will help you have more veins popping out!).

Ideally, you'll want to use a weight you would normally use for about 12 to 15 reps (depending on the exercise and get at least 20+. You're just going to do one set of that, so they'll be no reason to hold back.

The idea is to hammer out as many reps as you possibly can.

Then you'll rest 15 to 20 seconds, to flush out some of the lactic acid so that the burn doesn't hold you back on the NEXT part...stretch-focused sets.

You'll be immediately doing a set of 4 to 6 reps on a stretch-focused exercise for that muscle group, e.g. flyes for chest. Hold that bottom stretch position for at least 5 seconds on every rep. You'll want to use a fairly light weight on these as the goal is massive STRETCH not ego.

The idea behind this is to use the first set to fill the blood with muscle and then immediately use this stretch set to stretch fascia (the connective tissue "pillowcase" that surrounds the muscles). This fascia is critical for keeping the muscle contained but it's also tight enough to prevent the muscle from growing.

Think of it like a pair of tight jeans. When you get them out the laundry, you put them on then to loosen them up, you squat down a few times to stretch them out a bit. THAT is what we're trying to do with the stretch exercises here...stretch out those tight jeans.

You'll be doing this for every single body part...basically 1 "superset" of these two exercises.

DAY 2

On Day 2 of the training, you'll be doing almost the same thing. The only difference is that the first exercise is going to be 100 reps per set. You'll use very light weight and try and get 100 reps straight through in one set.

This very high rep training is ideal for building type 1 muscle fibers (slow-twitch endurance fibers) but that isn't the major goal...the major goal is increasing mircocirculation to the muscles.

The tiny blood vessels in your body where nutrient and oxygen exchange take place are known as capillaries. Our goal with 100 rep training is to increase the capillary density in your muscles so more nutrients and oxygen can reach the muscle fibers.

One of the major things that can hold back muscle development is lack of nutrients reaching the muscles. Think about the muscle groups you have the hardest time developing. They're the ones that are the hardest to get a pump in, right?

That means poor circulation and THAT is what we're going to fix with this style of training.

So you'll aim for 100 straight-through reps here. If you can't get to 100 all at once, get as many as you can then stop, set down the weight and take 10 seconds rest. Now pick up the weight and get as many more reps as you can.

Keep going until you reach 100 total reps. The short breaks will allow you to clear a bit of lactic acid while regenerating a bit of

ATP to help you keep going.

It's important to keep track of how much weight you're using and how many reps you got because the next time you do the 100 rep sets, you'll have two choices.

1. If you got 100 reps straight-through on that exercise, increase the weight by the smallest amount possible and use that weight this time.

2. If you didn't get 100 reps straight-through, repeat with the same weight. When you are able to get 100 reps, THEN you can increase the weight. You have to earn it.

You're also going to be doing the stretch-focused sets immediately after the 100 rep sets (15 to 20 seconds rest between the two), in order to achieve more fascial stretching.

On a side note, this type of training can make you VERY sore. I'd recommend taking 500 mg of Vitamin C a little before training. It can actually really help decrease soreness. That'll be a good thing because you're going to be doing heavy partials very soon!

Day 4 and 5 - Heavy Partial Training

Partial training is going to target the structure of your body as well as the nervous system. We'll be using supra-maximal weights in order to load the bones and connective tissue to prepare your body for heavier training.

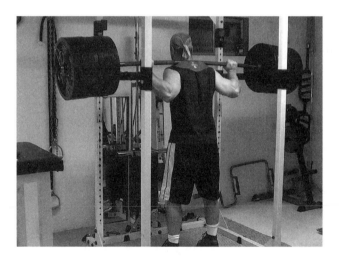

The much higher loads you'll be using will also help train the nervous system to fire more efficiently. It's a great combination that really helps increase the loads you're able to lift in full-range movements.

If you don't have access to a power rack, you can also use lighter loads but for higher reps and still get a good portion of the same benefits. For example, if you're doing partial bench press and you don't have a rack, I would NEVER recommend using a weight that's heavier than your max.

You're basically going to be doing very short range of motion in just the very strongest ranges of motion of various exercises. For example, the top few inches of the squat, bench press and deadlift will allow you to use large amounts of weight...a good amount higher than you can use for full range reps.

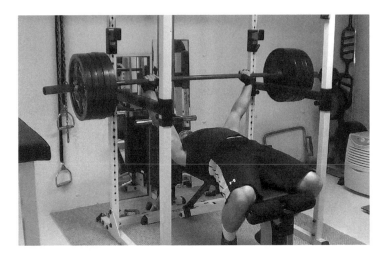

This increased loading is going to really thicken up your tendons and ligaments to be able to handle heavier loads without any problem.

Tip: Hold the lockout positions at the top of each lift for a 5 count. Holding that heavy weight really maximally loads the bones, muscles and connective tissue.

Alternatives to Heavy Partial Training

There are a variety of reasons why a person may not be able to do heavy partial training ranging from past injuries to equipment (lack of a power rack, for example).

In cases like this, I recommend still doing partial training but with VERY high reps instead. You'll use sub-maximal weights (relatively close to your 1 rep max) but for a LOT of reps.

For example, with bench press, instead of doing lockouts with 500 lbs for 5 or 6 reps, you would do 275 lbs for a set of 50+ reps. Use a fairly fast movement, since the weight is much lighter. The range of motion is the same.

This will help take the load off your body. The weight used will still providing good work for the connective tissue and the structure of your body, because you're still using a heavy load for a lot longer than you could with full-range reps.

In terms of safety, this means if you don't have a rack, you'll be able to do partial training without a problem. Just use the same set-up as you would for full-range reps.

SAFETY

IMPORTANT! Whenever you do bench press, you should have a spotter, unless you're doing them in the power rack.

This is especially important with partial training (and heavy lockouts in particular) because of the loads involved. DO NOT do heavy lockouts outside of a power rack. It's an accident waiting to happen.

When doing partials, always make sure and work your way up in loads gradually. Don't suddenly pile on a ton of weight when your body is not accustomed to it. By gradually building up, you'll make better strength gains and prevent injury.

Safety is also very important with fascial stretch-focused sets. Since you'll be holding the stretch position under load, you want to be sure you don't overstretch your joints. Don't try and go directly into the full stretch position all in 1 second.

Get close, then let your muscles sink into it, letting the resistance do the work.

Above all, know your limits and don't push yourself to the point of injury. No set you do in the gym is worth an injury that keeps you out of the gym. This is especially important with training techniques you might not be familiar with like the techniques found in this book.

They're all perfectly safe when done properly and with proper equipment.

Cluster Training

Cluster Training is extremely effective for producing a strong hypertrophy (muscle-building) stimulus in the body.

What is Cluster Training?

In a nutshell, it's a rep strategy that will allow you to take a weight you can normally only do 10 reps with and do it for more than 20 reps. The increase in time under tension on the muscles is extremely effective for forcing hypertrophy (muscle growth).

You avoid chemical fatigue (caused by lactic acid buildup) for longer, which helps you achieve fiber fatigue, which is more effective for actual growth.

The best way to explain Cluster Training is by example.

> 1. Start with a weight that you can do for 10 reps.
>
> 2. Do that weight for 4 reps.
>
> 3. Set the weight down and rest 10 seconds.
>
> 4. Pick up the weight and do 4 more reps.
>
> 5. Rest 10 seconds.
>
> 6. Repeat this until you've done 6 mini-sets of 4 reps with the weight

This sequence is one Cluster Set. It doesn't sound that hard but by the time you've finished the set (and your muscles will be screaming as you get near the end), you will have done 24 reps with a weight you normally could only do 10 reps with.

And this is not the only type of "clusters" you can do. You can very easily use 2 rep or even 5 rep "mini-sets", change up the short rest periods and adjust the number of mini-sets you're doing.

It could look like:

> 2 reps, 5 sec rest, for 10 sets
>
> 3 reps, 10 sec rest for 3 sets
>
> 5 reps, 10 sec rest for 3 sets

How It Works:

It's very simple - resting for 10 seconds between each mini-set of 4 reps allows your body to clear out some of the waste products accumulated by the training. This allows you to reach true muscular failure through tension on the muscles rather than by waste product accumulation forcing you to stop.

It's somewhat similar to rest-pause training, if you're familiar with that, but instead of taking each set close to failure, your goal is to delay fatigue and complete all the mini-sets.

It's a powerful technique that digs right at the heart of muscle hypertrophy. Working the fibers in this fashion provides a tremendous stimulus for muscle growth, even under lower-calorie conditions.

Notes:

- It will take you a few times through to properly judge how much weight to use in specific exercises. If you have to quit before completing the 6 sets of 4 reps, simply reduce the weight a little next time. If you make it through all the 6 sets or 4 reps easily, you can either stay where you are at (fatigue will catch up to you) or increase the weight next time if the weight was way too easy.

- Use good form on all reps. If you have to cheat to get the reps, you will lose tension in the target muscles when the idea is to generate maximum tension. You'll get more out of the technique by keeping your form tight. If you can't get to 4 reps, end at wherever you need to end, be it 2 or 3 reps. You've got 10 seconds till your next try at it.

Nick Nilsson

- Be strict with your 10 second intervals. The best way is to have a partner count it out for you or have a timer to keep you honest. Those 10 seconds can go by very quickly when you're on your 5th set of squats. Do your very best to keep up.

- You can choose to do all your Cluster Training sets using the same exercise or mix up your exercises (not during the

- Cluster set itself, however, only from one round to the next).

- This type of training will also enhance the carbohydrate loading you are also doing during this time, if you're using the Low-Carb Option. Intense training has been shown to increase glycogen uptake in the muscles as it relates to carb loading [Reference #5]. So performing this style of training will not only help increase muscle mass, it will help stimulate your body to load up on nutrients as well.

Pyramid Cluster Training

This is Cluster Training with an increasing and decreasing rep scheme. This technique allows for greater weight to be used while still getting more reps than you normally could. Select a weight you could normally rep 5 or 6 times.

> **First set - 1 rep - rest 10 seconds**
>
> **Second set - 2 reps - rest 10 seconds**
>
> **Third set - 3 reps - rest 10 seconds**
>
> **Fourth set - 2 reps - rest 10 seconds**
>
> **Fifth set - 1 rep - done**

The first two sets are going to be relatively easy. The third set will be challenging to complete. The fourth and fifth sets will be tough but because you're also decreasing the reps on each set of those, you should be able to complete those as well.

This is a very challenging technique and **very** effective for building strength in a Cluster Training framework. In the Cluster Training part of the program, we'll be utilizing this style of training on the second two days of the training, using the more hypertrophy-oriented "normal" type training for the first two days.

Single Rep Cluster Training

This style takes Cluster Training to it's very base level...doing 1 rep at a time using about 90% of your maximum, for multiple sets with short rest.

The short rest allows you just enough time to regenerate some ATP...enough to get another rep. You'll keep hitting single reps with short rest for a number "sets", allowing you to do much more training load than you normally would be able to do in one normal set.

An example using bench press: if you can bench 300 lbs for 1 rep, put between 265 to 275 lbs on the bar. Do 1 rep, rack the bar and rest 10 seconds. Unrack and do 1 rep, then rest 10 seconds. Repeat these 1 rep sets for 10 to 12 reps. You can also increase the percentage of your one rep max and use about 95%, hitting a range of about 5 to 7 mini-sets.

This will allow you to get more reps of that near maximal weight than you could if you had to go straight through. This is GREAT for targeting the high-power fast-twitch muscle fibers that have the most potential for growth.

It's also going to train your nervous system to operate more efficiently when using near maximum weight...practice makes perfect! The more you practice with relatively heavy weight, the better you will be at lifting it.

When people go from doing 10 to 12 rep sets and then try and max out, they're body isn't prepared for that in a number of ways. The nervous system doesn't know how to fire all the muscle fibers at once because it's never had to. The connective tissue and muscles aren't used to near-max loads so injury can result.

This style of training does a tremendous job of preparing the body for heavy lifting and max attempts.

Bottom-Start Single Rep Cluster Training

This type of Cluster Training is done exactly the same as I described only with one major difference...instead of doing the exercises as you normally would, e.g. unrack the bench press bar, press it, then rerack it, you will instead start at the **BOTTOM** of every movement, from a dead stop.

The idea of this is to completely eliminate elastic tension from the muscles so they don't get ANY help out of the bottom of the exercises. Yes, we're trying to make things HARDER.

And by making things harder, you're going to get better results.

Using the bench press as an example, you will set the rails in the rack so that the bar is just slightly above your chest when you slide yourself under it. You'll get your body nice and tight then press the weight up from the rails from a dead stop. This forces your <u>muscles</u> to be responsible for the ENTIRE weight.

I've found doing this type of training in "single rep cluster" fashion to be extremely effective for building strength because not only does it take away the elastic assistance, the brief rest in between every rep allows you to reset your body into the ideal position before starting the next rep.

This helps keep you stronger, longer by allowing you to use perfect form on EVERY rep.

Going back to bench as the example, before you start each rep, you will squeeze your shoulder blades behind your back, get your knees bent and feet on the floor so that you can exert power with your legs. You'll get your elbows into the tucked position and you'll puff your chest out. You don't to have unrack the bar and potentially mess up your body position.

THEN you'll press the weight up and lower it back down. Then you'll take a few seconds rest then set yourself up again.

This works great for a variety of exercises...bench press, squats, front squats, barbell shoulder press, lying tricep extensions, close grip bench, dips (you can stand on the floor and do the rest). The reason I don't mention deadlifts is because you're ALREADY doing this technique with deadlifts when you lift the barbell off the floor on each rep - doing deadlifts like a "normal" exercise would mean starting at the TOP, lowering the weight then coming back up again.

Overall, this technique offers a LOT of potential and makes sure that you're training the MUSCLES and not just using elastic force to help yourself. Start conservative on the weight until you know your strength levels from a dead stop - it can be an eye-opener if you've never done this before.

Time/Volume Training

Time/Volume Training is a form of Density Training that accomplishes overload of the muscles through increasing training volume and workload within a specific timeframe (i.e. training density) rather than by directly increasing intensity. This approach uses lighter loads and keeps you away from muscular failure, which keeps the nervous system fresher.

This is a very structured form of Density Training that tells you exactly how many reps to do, exactly when to increase rest periods and exactly when to increase loads. There is ZERO guesswork and it doesn't force you to break your focus in order track your reps during your time periods.

How To Do It:

You can use this technique with just about ANY exercise, including bodyweight training. For mass-building purposes, it's going to be the most effective when done with the big, basic exercises, of course.

With bodyweight training, obviously you won't be able to choose your weight, but choose a version of that exercise that allows you to get at least 10 reps. For example, if you can do close-grip pull-ups for 12 reps but can only do wide-grip pull-ups for 6 reps, use the close grip pull-ups.

When using this technique with non-bodyweight, free weight exercises, use a weight you could normally get about 10 to 12 reps with on a "regular" set.

So here's how it works in a 15 minute interval...

- First, start by doing a set of 3 reps. You'll obviously be nowhere near failure on this first set. Now **stop and rest 10 seconds**. Now do another set of 3 reps. Stop and rest 10 seconds.

- Keep going using 3 rep sets and 10 seconds rest until you can't get 3 reps anymore. When this happens and you get to a set where you do 2 reps and you feel like it would be a struggle to get that third rep, THAT is your cue to stop. When you hit this point, begin taking **20 SECOND** rests in between your 3 rep sets.

- Keep going using 3 rep sets and 20 second rest until you again can't get 3 reps anymore. **Then take 30 SECOND rests** in between your 3 rep sets. If you have to increase again, go to 40 seconds, and so on.

- Keep going in this fashion until your 15 minutes are up.

It's just that simple! Basically, the idea here is not to go to failure on any of your reps but to manage your fatigue so that you can maximize your training volume (i.e. more reps and sets).

This training style does what's known as "**front loading**" your training...basically doing more work while you're fresher then moving to doing less work as you get fatigued. When it comes to volume-based training, this is THE best way to go.

You'll find when using this technique with different exercises (especially bodyweight exercises, where some tend to be a bit easier than others), you'll be able to go longer before having to increase rest periods. For example, when doing pull ups, you'll probably have to increase rest sooner than you will with push-ups.

But rest assured, even if you can do 50 push-ups, you'll STILL get to a point where you're not able to do 3 rep sets on 10 second rests and you'll have to bump up the rest periods.

It's a great way to work bodyweight exercises without resorting to high-rep endurance training. With the 3 rep sets, you're still hitting the power-oriented muscle fibers, which is what allows you to make this type of training work for mass building.

Take a few minutes in between body parts for recovery. Here are the time intervals for this type of training:

Back, Chest and Thighs	15 minute blocks each
Hamstrings, Shoulders, Biceps, Triceps, Calves and Abs	7 1/2 minute blocks each

A technique I like to use with calves and abs is to combine them both into one block, basically go back and forth between exercises, e.g. calf raises to abdominal sit-ups, with no rest in between. The time it takes to do a set of abs is your rest time for your calves, since they're totally different body parts that have nothing to do with each other.

When to Increase the Weight:

I have a VERY simple rule for increasing the weight. If you can make it 1/3 of the way through the time period while keeping to the 10 second rest periods, then increase the weight the next time you train that exercise.

For example, if you're bench pressing 185 lbs and you're able to keep doing 3 rep sets with 10 seconds rest for at least 5 minutes, then next time, put 195 lbs on the bar.

If you're doing barbell curls, you'll need to get past the 2 1/2 minute mark in order to increase the weight. If you DON'T reach that 1/3 mark, then just keep the weight exactly where it is.

It's a very easy, very natural way to gauge your progress because you have to EARN your loads. If you don't make the time then you don't increase the weight... simple as that.

Rest-Pause Training

R est-Pause Training is one of the most effective methods for really fully stimulating muscle growth. To do Rest-Pause Training, you basically do as many reps as you can with a specific weight, set the weight down for a short period of time, then immediately try and get as many more reps as you can.

That's the SIMPLE version of it. It's simple yet very effective.

To build the most muscle you'll want to use exercises that work the most muscle mass, like squats, deadlifts, split squats, bench press, shoulder-press, bent-over rows, barbell curls, dips, close-grip presses, stiff-legged deadlifts, etc.

In the *Mad Scientist Muscle* program, here's how you'll be doing Rest-Pause Training.

- Set a weight on the bar that you can hit about 10 reps with (there will be other training days that start at lower rep ranges - 5 reps). Do as many reps as you can with it and DO NOT go to failure. Stop a rep short of that do-or-die rep.

- Now rest 20 seconds.

- Do another set of as many reps as you can with that same weight, same exercise. It may be 3 to 5 reps here.

- Rest 20 seconds.

- Do a final set of as many reps as you can with that weight. It may only be 1 or 2 reps here.

- Take your prescribed rest in between rest-pause sets.

- Done. Sounds like not very much in terms of training volume but just wait until you try it!

When the program says 3 rest-pause sets, you will count one set as [work, rest 20 seconds, work, rest 20 seconds, work]. That's one set. Then you repeat the sequence 3 times with your prescribed rest in between.

When you're using the lower-rep start (5 reps), your first set will be 5. Your second set will probably be 2 or 3 and your third set will be 1 or 2 reps.

Notes on Rest-Pause Training:

- Don't go to complete failure on ANY part of the training. You want to stay a rep or two shy of a maximum effort in order so you don't trash your nervous system. Believe me, even a rep or two short of failure will work you HARD by the end of the set.

- You MUST strive to increase the weight you use on the exercises every time you do the same exercise again. For example, if you did 225 x 10 on the deadlifts one week, add 5 to 10 lbs onto that the next week. We're trying to force the progressive resistance in order to increase the workload on the muscles.

- You'll notice that the schedule does not call for squats the day after doing deadlifts. Because both of those exercises are so demanding on the entire body, doing both exercises in two days will be too much to recover effectively from.

- As with any program, you should do a warm-up before jumping in and doing the heavy work. Personally, I do a few lighter sets of the exercise I'm about to do as well as some general warm-up movements - you may need a more thorough warm-up for yourself, however. Save the static stretch for after your training, when your muscles are very warm and full of blood.

Triple Add Sets

The Triple Add Set is very a tough style to do but very effective. You will be hitting all three major muscle fiber types (I and

IIa IIb) as you go through the sets as well as pushing the limits of your strength with the very low reps.

To fully understand the effectiveness of the Triple Add Set, let's take a look at the muscle fiber types and why it's such a good thing to work all three of the major types at once.

- **Type I muscle fibers** are endurance-oriented muscle fibers. They primarily work in higher rep ranges and during aerobic exercise.

- **Type IIa muscle fibers** work when the weight used is moderate-to-heavy. This fiber type is most active in moderate rep range weight training (e.g. 5 to 10 reps per set)

- **Type IIb muscle fibers** are the explosive muscle fibers. They are called upon when the weight is very heavy and great power or explosiveness is needed.

When you lift a weight, your body recruits a certain number of muscle fibers to get the job done. It recruits a certain percentage of each type of fiber, depending on how heavy the load is. For instance, the lighter the load, the more Type I fibers will be called upon. The heavier the load, the more Type IIa fibers will be called upon. With very heavy loads, Type IIb fibers will be the most heavily recruited.

With regular training, your body learns to become more efficient with this recruitment and tries to get away with firing as few fibers as possible to get the job done. It's the body's natural tendency to conserve energy.

Unfortunately, this also leaves many muscle fibers underworked and not developed to their full potential. We need to find a way to force your body to recruit every available fiber to maximally work the muscle and develop it to its full potential. That's where the Triple Add Set comes in.

If you're familiar with Triple Drop Sets (where you start with a heavy weight for the first part, then drop to a lighter weight for more reps then drop to a somewhat lighter weight for more reps to finish with) then you're familiar with the basic idea of this style of training.

However, here's the switch: instead of starting with a heavy weight and working down, we're going to start with a light weight and work our way up.

The Triple Add Set technique will first exhaust your Type I muscle fibers with light weights and high reps.

Then it will work on the Type IIa muscle fibers by moving to heavier weights and moderate reps. Since Type I fibers are still being activated at this point, even though the weights are heavier, your body will still recruit more and more of those Type I fibers as you keep going.

On the third and final part of the set, very heavy weights will be used. Your Type IIb fibers will now be preferentially activated. But now, because the load is extremely demanding, your Type I fibers and even more of your Type IIa fibers are being recruited to help.

By the time you're done with the Triple Add Set, you've recruited almost every available muscle fiber in the target muscle. Then we do one or two more sets just to be sure they're completely worked.

How To Do It:

- Start with a light weight and do a high-rep set, e.g. 20 to 30 reps. Your muscles will be burning. This will hit the Type I endurance muscle fibers and fill the muscle with blood.

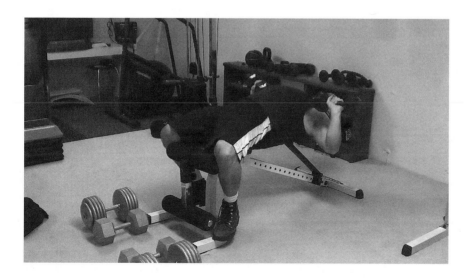

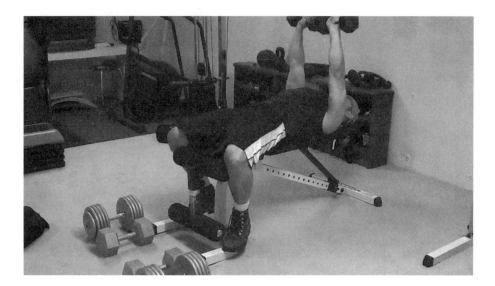

- Rest 10 seconds to flush out enough waste products in the muscles for you to keep going. This is basically the time it takes to switch weights on the machine or grab a new set of dumbbells.

- Next, you'll move on to a somewhat heavier weight and aim for about 6 to 8 reps. This will hit the Type 2 muscle fibers.

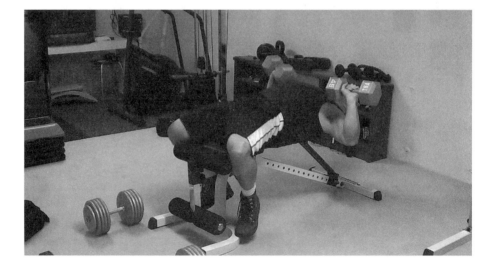

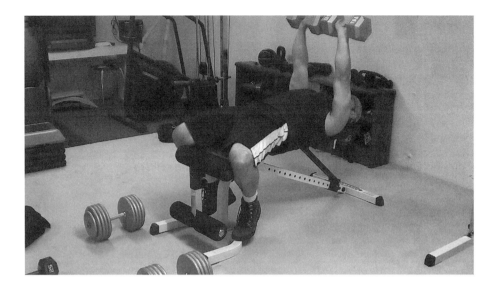

- Take 10 seconds rest again.

- After that, you will do your last set with a heavy weight, going for only 1 to 3 reps. This will work on strength and connective tissue.

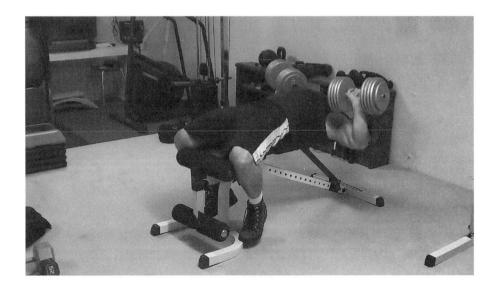

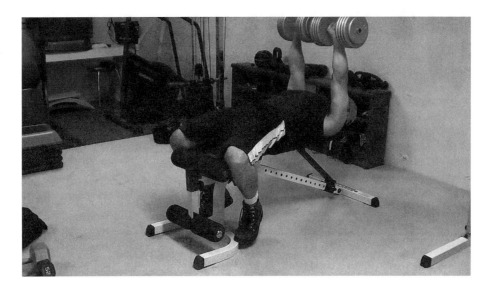

Your muscles will feel incredibly hard and pumped up. The effect of this type of training is immediately noticeable and very powerful.

It may take a little practice to figure out what weights you'll be using. It will really depend on how well your body deals with lactic acid buildup. This is a training stimulus your body will most likely NEVER have experienced before.

The first part of the set should use a very light weight. Go for strict form and go for the burn. The first time through you should get at least 20 to 30 reps or more. On the second add set, your reps will go down significantly as the waste products of the first set will not have been completely cleared yet.

The second part of the set should use about double what you used on the first part, e.g. start with 25 pound dumbbells then do 50 pound dumbbells (this increase will vary a lot depending on the exercise - experiment with the weights you use to find out what works for you).

The third and final part of the set is the hardest. Since you've already worked hard on the previous two parts, you will be using a weight that is lighter than what you'd normally use for this rep range in regular sets. When you do the third part, you will feel an extremely strong and deep burning in the muscles. You are tapping muscle fibers that have rarely been worked. The first two parts worked the majority of your fibers - every fiber you've got now has to kick in and fire to move the weight.

It's extremely hard and extremely effective. You'll either love it or dread it!

Low-Rep Strength Training

Building muscle goes hand-in-hand with building strength. After all, why would you want to LOOK strong but not BE strong?

This training style is all about strength. Low-reps are ideal for building strength along with the Type 2 muscle fibers that respond best to heavy loads and power-oriented lifting.

We'll be doing very straightforward strength-training here...3 sets for each body part consisting of 5 reps, then 3 reps then 1 rep, increasing the weight along with each decrease in reps.

When it comes to strength training, it can be really easy to overcomplicate things and make it actually LESS effective, which is why we're taking a very simple approach here.

No set should be taken to failure...keep that do-or-die rep in you on every set. It's easy for the nervous system to get overtaxed with heavy training and pushing to failure on heavy sets is a surefire way to actually set your strength gains BACK.

If you can't make the full 5 or 3, then just keep the weight the same on your next set. For example, if you get 4 reps instead of 5, just keep that same weight for your 3 rep set.

If you get to five and feel like you could do more. STOP. Don't do more. Just increase the weight a little more than you were planning to on your 3 rep set.

On your one rep sets, keep in mind that while it's just for a single rep, we're not trying to do a true one rep max test here. You should be at about 95 to 98% of your 1 rep max, but not right at it.

We want to keep the nervous system relatively fresh with this training, focusing on loading the body with heavy weight, allowing it to get use to training heavy. Towards the end of the deload week, THAT is when you're going to try and hit a 1 rep max!

Off/Deload/Fun/Strength Test

This is one of the most CRITICAL weeks of the training program...and it doesn't involve a whole lot of training. This is known as a "deload" in that we're greatly backing off on the amount of training that we're doing... almost completely off in this case.

This week is broken up in to three main sections...Off, Fun and Strength Test. I'll go through each one in detail below.

1. Off

Taking time off hard, heavy training is extremely important for making long-term gains in muscle size. When you train continuously with weights, your body doesn't get a chance to fully repair itself...the muscles, the connective tissue, the nervous system...even just mentally, you need the break.

Taking time out of the gym is going to help prevent burnout and actually give you better results in the long term by giving your body a chance to recover.

That's why I'm purposefully FORCING you to take time and building it right into the program. DO NOT skip this week and go right into the next cycle. I know if you're making good gain, it'll be tough to back off but trust me. Your body needs it even if you don't think it does.

When you track it from the last day of the "Intensification" phase, you'll have at least 4 days completely off and out of the gym. Feel free to just rest completely or to do other less intense physical activities that you enjoy.

2. Fun

On one of the days, I have a day labeled "Fun." This is a completely optional day...if your body is still feeling beaten up from the previous training you've done, you can take this day completely off and just relax.

Otherwise, if you want to get back into the gym, we're going to take this day to work on some fun exercises.

For example, if you love Concentration Curls, you're not going to be really doing any of those in the main program because they're just not good mass builders. Now's your chance to do them.

I'm also going to include a number of unique ones that you can mess around with and have some fun with, too.

Basically, this day is all about having some fun with your training...don't push too hard. We're still trying to deload and ease up on your body a bit. These "fun" exercises will give your body some unique movement patterns to keep things interesting.

The next day is going to be completely off again before we go to the Strength Test day.

3. Strength Testing

Feedback on your progress is extremely important and your strength is one of THE best gauges (besides increases in size and scale weight) for determining if your training is moving in the right direction.

True One Rep Max testing is demanding, which is why we only do it once per cycle...we're doing near max training during some phases of the cycle, which will help prepare your body for the One Rep Max testing we do on this day, but because this one is all about performance, we want to only do 1 hard set (maybe 2 or 3 if you feel you have more in you) per exercise, your One Rep Max lift.

Be very sure you keep track of your One Rep Max lifts so you can chart your progress as you move through the different cycles. If you see one cycle working better for you than others, you can go back more frequently to it to maximize your results.

When doing max lifts, use whichever exercise you most want to determine a true max for FIRST. Because the lifts you do after that may not be a true maximum, given the effort you put into the first one. So if you really want to know your max bench, do that first.

I've included instructions on how to do a One Rep Max lift, including the full ramp-up and how to use feeler sets to determine the load you're going to go for. It's critical you don't fatigue yourself by doing too much as you lead up to the your One Rep Max lift but you also want to be sure you're preparing your muscles and connective tissue and joints for the maximal loads.

4. When You're Done, What Comes Next?

After you've completed your Strength Test day, you've got two choices. 1.) Continue with a different cycle of the *Mad Scientist*

Muscle program or 2.) Move on to a different program, for fat loss, strength or muscle-building.

This program is put together in two month blocks specifically for this reason and therefore you don't have to make a huge commitment to this program in order to see great results.

Each two month block stands alone and is designed to take you through a full up and down cycle of Accumulation and Intensification.

What comes next is up to you!

Aerobic Interval Training

I'll be honest with you; cardio training can go either way on a muscle-building program. For people who have good recovery, adding in some cardio can help keep body fat levels in check and help maintain cardio capacity.

For others, every little bit of energy not devoted to the muscle-building process is a drain on their reserves and can set them back.

This is why I've included cardio training sessions in the program but they're completely OPTIONAL and not very frequent. It's up to you to determine whether you feel you'll benefit from the addition of cardio or not.

To that end, here are my thoughts on cardio training in this muscle-building program.

1. It should be done with an eye on minimizing its impact on overall recovery.

This means we're NOT going to be doing high-intensity sprint interval training. My recommendation is Aerobic Interval Training (which I'll talk about in more detail below), which doesn't impact muscle recovery to any great extent and still carries better cardiovascular benefits than long-duration, straight-through cardio training.

Higher intensity interval training is totally fine IF getting in better cardio shape is your major goal or if you're on a fat-loss program. Since this program is about NEITHER of those things, we won't be doing that type of training.

2. The Accumulation phases of this program call for ever-increasing training volume with decreasing rest periods.

The practical upshot of this is that for much of the program, you'll be getting a good cardiovascular workout just from the weight training alone.

How To Do Aerobic Interval Training:

This type of interval training involves relatively long work periods and shorter rest periods. Work periods, for our purposes, are 2 to 4 minutes long in this type of training. The idea is not to take it easy for that work time but to work at a speed that challenges you to be able to make it to the end of that work interval. Your 2 minute interval pace is, therefore, going to be significantly faster than your 4 minute interval pace.

Nick Nilsson

The rest interval for this type of training is between 30 seconds to a minute. Naturally, the shorter the rest period, the tougher the training will be. Too much rest will allow your body to recover too much, lessening the overall training effect of the exercise.

Here are some examples of a number of different intervals you can use in your training:

Work	Rest
2 min.	30 sec.
4 min.	1 min.
3 min.	45 sec.
2 min.	1 min.
4 min.	30 sec.

When using these intervals, you can choose to stick to the same time intervals (e.g. do 2 minutes hard and 30 seconds slow for the duration of the workout) or mix it up with different time intervals as you go through your session. This type of training should be done for about 15 to 20 minutes.

The key thing to remember in terms of Aerobic Interval Training and muscle building is that we're not looking to push it to the max. Our goal here is MAINTAINING cardio conditioning, not killing ourselves to improve it.

The Core Combo

The Core Combo is very simple. It includes components designed to improve your abdominal and lower back strength, as well as the rotator cuff to keep your shoulders strong and healthy. These areas are CRITICAL for assisting with overall muscle development.

This combination is done to ensure that no muscles are underdeveloped. Generally, if a person does not do regular deadlifting or other direct lower back work, the lower back can easily become a weak link. This may lead to lower back pain and decrease the weight you can lift with exercises such as squats.

The Core Combo is done after almost every single workout (the exact times you will use the combo are listed in the program phases in the Appendix). The abdominal work will be targeted toward increasing overall core and ab strength rather than how your abs look (meaning, you're not going to be doing a lot of crunching type movements but exercises that target core stability).

Working the rotator cuff is VERY important in a strength and mass program. The four muscles of the rotator cuff (infraspinatus, supraspinatus, subscapularis, and teres minor) serve to stabilize the humerus (your upper arm bone) in the shoulder joint. When you do heavy bench pressing and shoulder pressing, rotator cuff strength is ESSENTIAL for keeping your shoulders healthy.

The Core Combo should take no more than five minutes or so to complete. You go from abs straight to lower back, straight to rotator cuff with minimal rest between sets (about 20 to 30 seconds).

Ab Exercises

Use any of the three ab exercises listed on the next few pages, or feel free to use your own. (Remember, I've chosen exercises targeted for core strength.) The number of sets is limited, so work them hard and make them count! Aim for six to 10 reps per set and go to failure. Rest about 30 seconds between ab sets. I would recommend using only one exercise in your ab sets to make setup easier.

To develop core strength that is useful in heavy training, the abs need to be pushed hard with good resistance, not with endless reps with very little weight. Don't be shy about pushing yourself hard when it comes to adding resistance to the exercises.

Lower Back Exercises

For the lower back, use an isolation exercise such as the regular hyperextension, the hyper crunch, or the reverse hyperextension. Since you'll be doing regular heavy deadlifting and stiff-legged deadlifts, the lower back will get plenty of heavy work.

You can do lower back work for higher reps with just bodyweight or add resistance (by holding a dumbbell or barbell plate), then use lower reps to build strength in the area. Rest 30 seconds between sets.

Rotator Cuff Exercises

The rotator cuff muscles are essential for keeping the shoulder joint strong and healthy. Working them regularly is important. I've included an exercise I call the Three-In-One Rotator Cuff Exercise. It combines several different cuff movements into one movement. It's effective and saves time while giving your rotator cuff a complete workout.

Do one arm at a time, and take no rest between sets for each arm, basically going back and forth between right and left arm. Do sets of 10 to 12 reps per arm and don't push this muscle group to failure. The idea is to strengthen but not exhaust. You don't need heavy weight for this exercise.

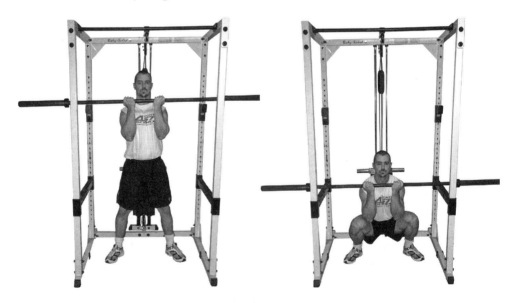

BarBell curl SquatS

Curl Squat

Why Is This Exercise So Effective?

This is an extraordinary exercise for building supporting strength and stability in the core muscles, especially for movements such as squats and deadlifts.

This exercise is simple to do with dumbbells, barbell, or cables. Each has its strengths and drawbacks, of course. The movement is similar to the front squat without any of the support you would normally get from your shoulders. All the support tension goes onto your abs!

The Barbell Version

Set the squat rack up so that the racks are one notch below where you would normally set them for squats. You do this because by the time you're done, it may be very hard to get the bar back to where you normally rack it. Set the safety rails just above where you normally set them for regular squats the first time you try this, too. When you develop a better feel for how it's done, you can lower them a little to get a fuller range of motion.

Step in front of the bar and hold it in the top position of the barbell curl. Now stand up, unracking the bar. Don't allow your elbows to brace against your midsection. This takes away from the supporting tension on the abs. Take a step back and get your feet set. Now, holding the bar in that top curl position through the entire movement, squat down as far as you can, then come back up. You don't actually curl the bar while doing the squat, you just hold it in the top curl position.

Hold your breath during the majority of this movement to keep greater stability in your core. Start holding as you start to go below the halfway point, and continue to hold it until you're about halfway back up. If you don't want to or are unable to hold your breath, exhale through pursed lips (as though you're blowing up a balloon). Keeping the breath held will maximize core stability and allow your abs to function more effectively during the movement. Since this exercise uses relatively light weight compared to a regular squat, holding your breath is not nearly as potentially dangerous. If you do feel lightheaded, rack the bar and rest.

Holding the resistance in front of your body, as you do in this exercise, takes away the shoulder support you would normally get with a front squat. The required supporting tension goes directly on the core muscles, which have to contract hard throughout the entire movement to keep the barbell from falling forward.

This exercise helps you get a feel for using the abs during a squat, which is extremely important for maximizing your squat strength. Using the abs while squatting does not come naturally and is very rarely taught or explained. But this exercise helps to greatly strengthen the abs for that specific purpose, making this a very powerful core and overall strength-building exercise.

When doing the exercise for the first time, start with just the bar, no matter how strong you are. This will help you get a feel for the movement, where to set the safety rails, and how far down you can comfortably go. When you're comfortable, work your way up slowly from there, as fatigue will come quickly. It's a movement your body will be totally unused to, no matter how many abdominal exercises you've done in your training career. The core muscles will tire before your legs do. Be sure to keep your lower back arched and tight while performing this movement.

If you are able to, go all the way down until your elbows touch your knees. This will give you the fullest range of motion. Tense the abs hard, especially at the bottom as you are coming back up. For extra resistance, pause at the bottom for a few seconds. This will give you the best feel for how the abs should be used when squatting.

With this exercise, holding the resistance in front of the body (like in a front squat) allows you to keep a more vertical body position. The tension will go onto the abs, but be aware that there will also be some tension to the lower back. Because you are holding the weight out in front of you, the lower back must also contract to help stabilize the spine. As you keep up with the exercise, your lower back will get stronger.

Another great benefit is that your breathing muscles (the intercostals) never get a chance to relax during this movement. From top to bottom and back up (even while you're "resting" at the top), your breathing muscles are being challenged by the weight they are being forced to support. This can build up great lung capacity and breathing strength (excellent for athletes who need great cardio capacity). And it carries directly over to your work capacity in the regular barbell squat.

The Cable Version

The cable version is essentially the same in form as the barbell version but with one big difference: The angle of the cable adds forward pulling resistance. This adds another tension to the abs because, in addition to supporting the weight, they're also forced to contract to keep you from falling forward. The exercise doesn't require as much stability control as the barbell version, however, and your breathing muscles won't be challenged as much.

Get the bar to the top of the curl position, take a step back, then perform the exercise as you would with the barbell.

If you have an adjustable-height cable setup, it's best to start this exercise with the pulley set a few notches up. (This makes it easier to get into the start position.) If you just have a low-pulley, you'll need to curl the weight up into position to start the movement.

The Dumbbell Version

The dumbbell version can be done two ways: with two dumbbells or with one. The execution with two dumbbells is exactly the same as with the barbell version, the only difference being that you have to curl or clean the weight up to the top of the curl position to do the exercise.

If you are using only one dumbbell, this one-sided tension will allow you to put torque on the abs to work the sides (switch sides with each set for a balanced workout). When you are using one dumbbell, you can also drop your elbow inside your knees to go down deeper. You can get your butt right down by your heels with this one. Very challenging!

Common Errors

1. **Doing this exercise after a bicep workout**As you can imagine, performing this exercise is not going be as effective if you've just finished a bicep workout. The biceps will already be fatigued, and you'll limit the amount of weight you can use and how long you can hold it. Use this exercise on non-bicep training days.

2. **Going too fast**Dropping down quickly in the squat will put extra stress on the biceps as you come up and reduce the tension on the abs. This exercise should be done very deliberately, with no bouncing or fast movements. If you have a tendency to do either, pause at the bottom for a few seconds to stop the bouncing.

3. **Using too much weight** Since the legs are so much stronger, it's tempting to use too much weight for this exercise. Remember, our goal here is NOT to work the legs or the biceps, but to work the abs. The legs and the biceps are only here to help push the abs. If your biceps fatigue before your abs get a good workout, you need to reduce the weight.

4. **Leaning forward** Try to keep your upper body as vertical as possible. It's very similar to a front squat. Having the weight in front of you allows you to stay vertical more easily. Leaning forward will cause the barbell to shift forward, which will put more tension on the biceps, causing them to fatigue prematurely. As you start to fatigue, you will notice you have a tendency to lean forward. This is because the supporting abs are weakening. Do your best to keep vertical. Once you start to move too far forward, end the set.

5. **Bar too close to collarbones** If the bar gets too close to the collarbones, you will lose some of the tension in the abs. Keep the bar at least a few inches away to maximize the supporting tension and torque demanded of the abs. If it comes too close, you may be tempted to rest the bar on your collarbones, which will turn it into an uncomfortable front squat.

6. **Letting the elbows brace strongly against the midsection** If you let the elbows press strongly into the midsection, you take away some of the tension on the abs. A little contact is fine, especially as you tire, but don't rely on using this technique or you make the exercise less effective. Letting the elbows sink in will also tend to hunch your back over, putting pressure on the lower back. This will pull your torso and center of balance forward, putting more tension on the biceps, making you dig the elbows in more! Keep the elbows out front, away from your body, and you'll keep a better body position and do a more effective set.

Tricks

1. **Look forward and slightly up** When you squat, keep looking forward and slightly up. This will help you keep an arch in your lower back and keep you from leaning forward. You want to avoid forward lean, as it causes the biceps to fatigue prematurely.

2. **Don't breathe too deeply in or out as you are coming down or pushing back up** Breathing too much during this exercise reduces core stability and can compromise form. For best core stabilization, keep your breath carefully controlled. At the bottom, you can hold your breath for a few

moments to get the most solid stability. As you come up, exhale through pursed lips after you've come about one-quarter to one-half of the way. This technique shouldn't be used if you have blood pressure issues, however, as it does cause an increase in blood pressure. Keep a careful eye on how you feel if you do choose to do this. If you feel any dizziness, end the set and don't use this technique the next set.

3. **Pause at the bottom** To really maximize the tension on the abs, pause for a few seconds at the bottom and focus on really squeezing and tightening your abs hard. As you start to come back up, try to push with your abs as well. This will help you feel what it's like to use the abs to help push out of the bottom when doing regular barbell squats.

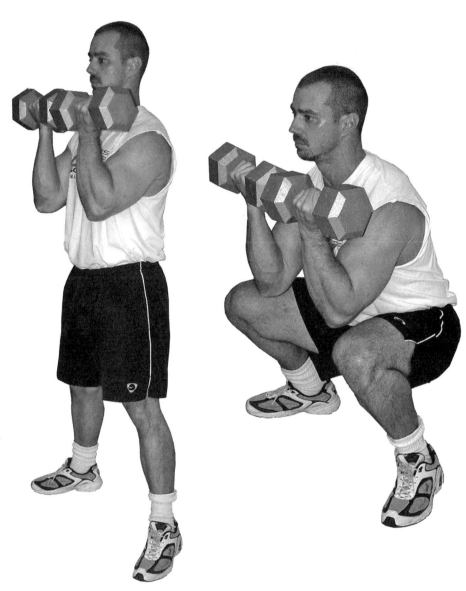

Dumbbell Curl Squats

Two-Dumbbell Ball Twist

Why Is This Exercise So Effective?

Using only a Swiss Ball and two dumbbells, you can achieve an extraordinary ab-tightening contraction around the entire midsection musculature. This exercise places great stretch, along with great tension, on the obliques, forcing quick abdominal development.

How to Do It

You need two dumbbells and a Swiss Ball (I tell you how to do this on a regular flat bench in the Tricks section below). A smaller-size ball is better for this exercise, though any ball will work.

Lie on your back with your knees bent and your feet fairly wide apart. You need a good base of support so you don't roll off to the side of the ball. Hold two equal-weight dumbbells at arms-length directly above you. Press them together while doing this exercise (if they're separated, they'll move around more, making the exercise less efficient). Start with fairly light dumbbells the first time you try this movement.

Keeping your head facing directly up/forwards and your hips horizontal, lower both dumbbells slowly and under complete control down to the left. Hold your breath and tighten your midsection as you come down to the fully twisted position. Prepare to push hard against the ground with your left foot to maintain your balance.

Your left arm is going to bend to about 90 degrees at the elbow as you lower the dumbbells to the side while your right arm should stay perfectly straight. Your upper body should stay in the same position on the ball—no rolling to the opposite side to compensate for the weight to the side. This torque is what makes the exercise so valuable. Bending your lower arm is critical to keeping your torso in the same position on the ball.

Because you are using two separate dumbbells, you create a very different stress on the abdominal area than any you've experienced before.

When you're at the bottom, your upper left arm will touch the surface of the ball. (Don't let it rest or lose tension at this point!) Reverse the direction by simultaneously pulling with your right side abs and pushing with your left side

Nick Nilsson

abs. The right arm movement is similar to a rear delt lateral, while the left arm movement is similar to a dumbbell press.

Remember to keep the dumbbells pressed together tightly. The opposing tension in the abs puts a lot of torque across the whole area. Be very sure you're not just pushing with the bottom arm but also pulling with the top arm.

Be sure not to bounce out of the bottom. Try to feel a stretch in the right side as you start the change of direction.

If you have any lower back pain issues, this exercise does put some stress on the lower back. If you do try it, go very light and take it very slowly.

Common Errors

1. **Separating the dumbbells** Keep them pressed together throughout the movement. If they separate, they're harder to control, and you disperse the tension on the abs.

2. **Rolling around on the ball** For best results, be sure to keep yourself as stationary as possible on the ball. If you roll to the side, you take some of the torque off the abs and lose effectiveness.

3. **Moving too quickly** This is NOT a ballistic exercise. There should be no bouncing or fast movements involved. Lower the dumbbells slowly to the sides and change direction very deliberately by using muscle power, not bouncing.

Tricks

1. **Change the arc** You can bring the dumbbells down at various angles to the torso to change where the exercise hits your abs. By bringing it down beside your head, you'll hit the upper area of your obliques. By bringing it down toward your hip, you'll hit the lower area. Just remember to always keep your head looking straight up and set your feet wide apart for the best base of support.

2. **Use a flat bench instead** You can also do this exercise on a flat bench. Instead of lying flat on the bench as you normally would for a bench press, you'll be resting only your upper back on the end of the bench.

   To get into this position, sit on the very end of the bench. Now move your butt off the bench and squat down in front of it. Lean back and place your upper back on the bench end. Keep your hips down and set your feet fairly wide apart.

This is the position you should maintain while doing the exercise. The bench is a more solid surface, and it is just as effective for the exercise. But there won't be any surface to make contact with the bottom arm as you lower the weight down. Keep an eye on how far down you go to the side. All other techniques still apply.

3. **Use a heavier weight** If you are using a heavy weight, you will need to shift your upper body somewhat to the other side of the ball in order to stay on the ball. The increased resistance will make up for it.

Be extra careful that the dumbbells don't separate. It is much harder to control heavier dumbbells if they do.

As you rotate back up, exhale through pursed lips to keep stability in your abs and so you don't pass out.

Push VERY hard with the same side leg as the weight is on. You'll need all the help you can get.

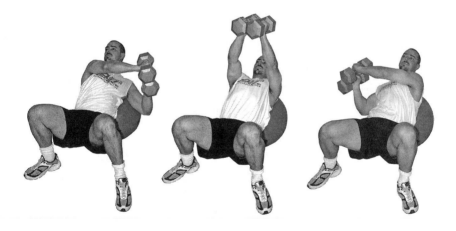

Two Dumbbell Ball Twists

Abdominal Sit-Up

Why Is This Exercise So Effective?

This is a sit-up movement that works the abs instead of the hip flexors. It will work all the muscles in your midsection in one exercise.

The standard crunch only addresses part of the function of the abdominals. This exercise targets the flexed (arched back) range of motion of the abs and uses the weight of your entire torso as resistance.

Lie on your back on the floor. Roll up a towel or mat and slip it beneath your lower back just above the waistband. (The size of the towel affects your body position during this movement; use a fairly large towel.).

Your knees should be bent about 90 degrees. Keep your feet close together and your knees fairly wide apart. This prevents the hip flexors from having a direct line of pull, minimizing their involvement. Do not anchor your feet or have someone hold them down. This automatically activates the hip flexors. You will get the most out of this exercise by minimizing their involvement.

The difficulty of this exercise depends on where you hold your hands. The hardest position is above your head at arms-length, then beside your head, then across your chest, then straight down between your legs or at your sides. Start with the easiest position first. Progress to the other positions as you get stronger.

You are now ready to crunch.

Keeping your torso straight and stiff, start the sit-up by tightening your lower abs. As you continue up, imagine trying to push your face up against the ceiling (think up, not around). When you reach about 25 to 30 degrees above horizontal, hold for a second and squeeze hard.

Keep your back in contact with the towel at all times and always maintain tension in the abs. Lower yourself down slowly and under control. Do not just drop back to the ground. The negative portion of this exercise is extremely effective.

Common Errors

1. **Using momentum** Do not swing yourself up to get started. Always squeeze yourself up using ab power. Start with the easiest positions first,

for example, arms down at your sides. If you are having trouble doing this exercise, try using a slant board (with your head higher up).

2. **Losing tension at the top** This occurs when you come too far up. Always maintain contact with the towel and keep tension in your abs.

3. **Allowing the glutes to come off the ground** Keep the glutes on the ground at all times. The glutes tend to come up at the start of the rep, when your abs are first trying to get your body off the ground and your back is pivoting over the towel.

4. **Coming up too far** This error actually takes tension off the abs just when they should be getting the most tension. Keep your lower back in contact with the towel throughout the exercise.

5. **Improper towel placement** The towel should be just above the waistband area in the small of the back. Placing it too high or too low will affect the exercise negatively.

Tricks

1. **Move your hand position through the set** When you get stronger at this exercise, start with your hands over your head. When you fail with that, continue with your hands beside your head, then continue with hands across the chest, then hands at your sides or between your legs to finish. It is a merciless drop set.

2. **Use extra resistance** Hold a weight plate in your hands. Start very light, say five to 10 pounds, as balance can be a problem, especially because your feet should not be anchored.

3. **Spot yourself** Extra resistance, as described above, can also be used to spot yourself. Hold the weight plate out in front of you instead of behind you. This will act as a counterbalance and help pull your body up.

4. **Use an extra hard contraction** This technique will give you an extra hard contraction: Once you come up to about 25 degrees, bring your arms in so your forearms are in front of your face (like a boxer covering up). Pivoting just below the rib cage using your upper abs only, crunch your elbows down toward your hips and squeeze hard, exhaling completely. Your lower abs will not move at all. This makes it look like a two-part movement: the sit-up, then stop, then the crunch over.

You can also give yourself a little spot by grabbing onto your legs and pulling over.

5. **Work the sides** To work the sides more during this movement, come up to 25 degrees. Then do a twisting crunch over to the side. Don't do the twist as you are coming up in the sit-up. Do it after you are up to about 25 degrees.

6. **Breathe at the top** Try holding the contraction at the top and breathing in and out a few times. This will really force your abs to contract.

7. **Lengthwise on a bench** Lie lengthwise along a bench with the towel under your lower back. Your shoulders should be just off the end of the bench so you can stretch back and down a little. The edge of the bench should be just below the shoulder blades. Your head and arms will be hanging off the end of the bench. This will give you a greater range of motion. Execute the movement the same way.

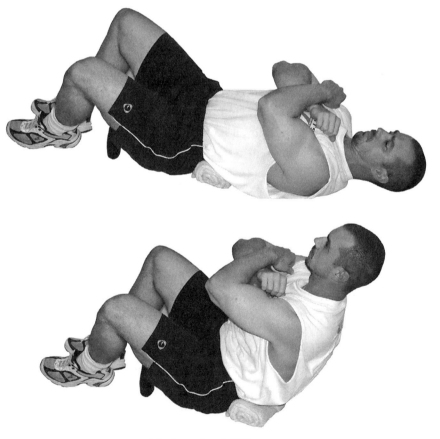

Abdominal Sit-ups

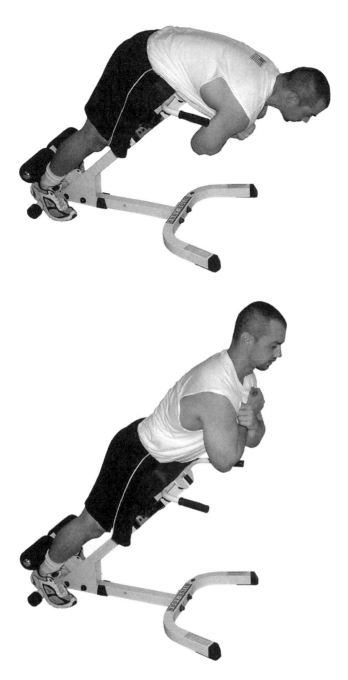

Hyper Crunch

Hyper Crunch

Why Is This Exercise So Effective?

This variation of the hyperextension is far more effective than the typical hyperextension for training the spinal erectors directly. The secret is not bending at the hips but flexing the spine at the vertebrae themselves.

It is better to have a rounded pad for this version. If you don't and the exercise is too uncomfortable, fold a mat and put it on top of the thigh pads.

Instead of resting your thighs on the pads, rest your midsection on the pads. The edge of the pad should be just under your rib cage rather than at the hips.

Suck in your gut for comfort. This is especially important on the way down. If you have a potbelly, this exercise may be uncomfortable. This exercise is NOT recommended if you are pregnant as you will not be able to position yourself on the bench safely. Stick to the regular hyperextension.

Crunch over the edge of the pad, rounding your lower back until your head is down. You can hold your hands crossed in front of your chest if you like.

Crunch back up using only the spinal erectors. This exercise uses only spinal flexion and extension, not hip flexion and extension, removing the glutes as a prime mover and using them only isometrically. Squeeze hard at the top and repeat.

The downside to this movement is that it can feel uncomfortable on the abdomen. It should not be done by those with large bellies. To ease pressure on the abdomen, inhale and exhale only at the top of the movement and suck in your gut during the movement.

Common Errors

1. **Not curling the abdomen over the bench** The major advantage of this exercise lies in curling the abdomen, i.e., flexing the spine, over the edge of the bench. If you don't flex the spine, you won't fully work the erector spinae muscles through their full range of motion.

2. **Using momentum** Never use momentum on any lower back exercise. This can be very dangerous as it places stress on the spine when it's in a vulnerable position.

Tricks

1. **Imagine extending one vertebra at a time as you come up** This imagery will help you activate the spinal erectors. When you visualize each one extending in a sequence, each of the small spinal erector muscles will fire in order. You can also visualize yourself curling your back around a ball to achieve the same effect.

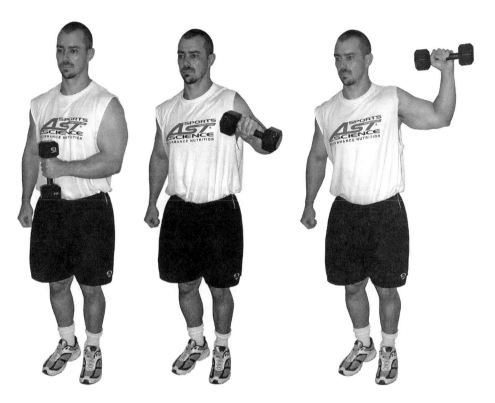

3 in 1 Rotator Cuff Raises

Nick Nilsson

Three-In-One Rotator Cuff Raise

Why Is This Exercise So Effective?

Maintaining a strong rotator cuff muscle group is essential for optimum shoulder stability and strength. This exercise combines aspects of three different rotator cuff exercises, improving your efficiency when you exercise your rotator cuff muscles.

Start in a standing position with your upper arm vertical, your forearm crossed in front horizontally, and your shoulder internally rotated.

Hold the dumbbell in front of your abdomen. This is similar to the start position of what is called the Lying "L" Raise (a common rotator cuff exercise), where you lie on your side on a bench. In this exercise, though, you are in a standing position.

During this entire movement, keep a constant 90 degree bend in your elbow.

Externally rotate and abduct your shoulder (raise your upper arm up and to the side while bringing the dumbbell up and back).

While you raise your upper arm to a horizontal position, raise your forearm to a vertical position.

This should be accomplished in a smooth motion.

This is a much more time-efficient method of working the rotator cuff, as you hit three basic types of rotator cuff movements in one movement.

Common Errors

1. **Throwing the weights up** Don't use momentum on this exercise. You will get far more out of it if you strive for slow, controlled movements, focusing on continuous tension. Throwing the weight up is just going through the motions. You might also injure the sensitive structures of the rotator cuff.

2. **Improper timing on the movement** The movement should be a smooth, balanced transition from one position to the other. Choppy or jerky timing will reduce effectiveness.

3. **Moving your upper body excessively** If you find your torso bobbing

forward and backward to get the weight up, you are using too much weight. This exercise is most useful when done with strict form and continuous tension. Be sure you aren't trying to heave the dumbbells.

Tricks

1. **Change where you start and finish the exercise** You can try an alternate starting position that will keep more tension on the shoulders. Instead of holding your forearms horizontal and the dumbbells directly in front of your abdomen, try to keep your forearms up and the dumbbells held just under your chin.

   You will almost look like a boxer in the guard position. The position also resembles the top position of a two-dumbbell hammer curl if you finish with the dumbbells just under your chin. When you start the movement, let the dumbbells dip down slightly before you swing them around and start the rotator cuff movement.

How to Max Out

Maxing out isn't just about throwing a lot of weight on the bar and seeing how much you can do. In order to get a REAL One Rep Max, you have to be thoughtful in your preparations leading up to your maximum attempt.

Above all, we don't want any injuries but secondarily, we don't want fatigue from excessive warm-ups to reduce your actual One Rep Max attempt.

You can do these lifts in any order but start with the one you most want to know your TRUE max on. The other lifts will probably be a little lower because of the effort you'll put in on the first attempt.

When doing max lifts, keep your body VERY tight. You want to be pushing/ pulling with maximum stability. This includes holding your breath. By holding your breath, you will have maximum stability. If you have high blood pressure, don't do it, but if you don't have blood pressure issues, holding your breath for the short time it takes to do one rep is going to give you added power and strength.

So after you've done a general "blood pumping" type warm-up, here's the sequence for maxing out...

Maxing Out on the Deadlift:

Say you're going to be aiming for a max attempt at 495 lbs, which is 5 plates. We don't want to immediately jump to that on the first or second set. We want to ramp up to it, waking up the nervous system and gradually preparing your body for heavier and heavier loads.

1. You'll want to start with one plate per side and do 5 or 6 reps. This is a very light warm-up set to get some blood pumping.

2. Since the first set was very light, you won't really need a rest here, just put 225 on the bar and do 3 more reps.

3. Rest about 30 seconds after you put 315 on the bar and do 2 or 3 reps. it's getting heavier now. Rest about a minute while you're loading the next weight level on.

4. Get 405 on the bar and do 1 rep. You'll notice that we're not doing a lot of reps at each level here, even with the light weight. The idea is to

wake up the nervous system while still gradually preparing the body for heavier loads. We're not trying to do a full workout here so DO NOT push yourself hard on any of these sets.

These previous sets are also what are called "feeler" sets. You'll use these lead-up sets to gauge how strong you're feeling and to decide on your actual max weight that you're going to use.

5. Take a minute and a half rest and put 40 more lbs on the bar and do 1 rep. This is closing in on your max numbers - it's heavy enough that your nervous system is prepared for maximum lifting but not quite at the max level that it'll fatigue you. It'll give you the best idea of your strength levels for that day, too, depending on how fast you get the bar up.

6. Take at least 2 to 3 full minutes rest AFTER loading your max attempt weight on the bar (so load the bar then start your timer).

7. Now GO FOR IT!

8. Once you complete the lift, you can gauge how it felt to see if you think you can go up a bit more. If you feel you have more in you, add it on and take at least 3 minutes rest before trying again.

Deadlift Notes:

The actual loads and number of ramping sets you'll be doing will depend on the amount of weight you're going to maxing out with. If your max deadlift is 275, you won't need as many sets to lead up to that. I would start with 135 lbs and do 3 to 4 reps, then use 185 and do 2 reps, then use 225 lbs and do 1 rep THEN go for your max.

When you're lifting heavy weights on deadlift, don't try and pop the bar off the ground all in one shot. You want to "squeeze" the bar off the ground.

What happens with heavy weight is that the bar bends. The first few inches of the pull are simply putting bend in the bar before the weight even comes off the ground. If you pop the weight off the ground, the weights will come up then they will bounce back DOWN, pulling the bar down with them.

Not so critical with lighter weight, but with a max, you don't want to have bouncing weights pulling down adding more resistance.

So first, pull the bend into the bar THEN pull the plates off the ground.

Maxing Out on the Bench Press

Generally speaking, the vast majority of people are going to be able to deadlift a fair bit more than they can bench press. So the ramping phase is shorter for benching than it is for deadlifting. I've found that it's also easier to fatigue your upper body with overdoing the warm-up than it is on the lower body so watch out.

1. If you're attempting a max bench of 315 lbs (3 plates), start with 135 on the bar and do 4 or 5 reps.

2. Rest about 30 seconds then go up to 225 lbs for 2 or 3 reps.

3. Rest about 90 seconds then go to 275 lbs for 1 rep.

4. Rest 2 to 3 minutes then go to your 315 lb max attempt.

5. When you complete the lift, if you feel you can go higher, load it on, take at least 3 minutes rest then go again!

Bench Notes:

If you're not doing bench press in a power rack, be ABSOLUTELY SURE you have a good spotter for your max attempt. NEVER max out on bench press without a spotter (heck, never push yourself right close to failure on bench press if you don't have a spotter! The last thing you want to do is be trapped under the bar).

Squeeze the bar HARD...so hard that your fingers turn blue, if you have to. This will increase nervous system activation. I've also found it useful to try and imagine like you're pulling the bar apart, to fire the triceps for assistance.

The most critical thing to remember is to NOT flare your elbows wide out to the sides. This puts more stress on the shoulders. Keep your elbows tucked in more to save shoulder stress - practice this in your training and make sure you do it on every rep.

Maxing Out on Squats:

The approach for the Squat is going to be pretty much the same as for the Deadlift, and it'll also depend on the amount of weight you're going to be using. Use the "feeler" sets and ramping up to gradually get your body used to using more and more weight.

With squatting in the power rack, one of the things to be aware of it stepping back out of the racks. When doing your squats in regular training, you should be practicing a minimalist approach to stepping back, two steps and that's it. This means no shuffling and taking 4 steps back.

You should unrack, take one step back with your left and one step back with your right, directly into squat stance position. You can get away with it when doing lighter weight but with a max attempt, you want to minimize the steps you take so that you're not fatiguing your legs unnecessarily.

Maxing Out on Other Lifts:

The big three lifts are the most common ones to max out on. Some exercises just aren't suited to single-rep maximum attempts, for example calf raises, pushdowns, incline dumbbell curls, leg curls, flyes, etc.

Some of the other exercise I have found useful to max out on are:

- Stiff-Legged Deadlifts

- Barbell Press or Barbell Clean and Press

- Weighted Chin-Ups

- Barbell Curls

- Close Grip Bench Press (flat or decline)

You can use the same ramping and feeler set techniques for these lifts as I talked about above. The key is to make sure you're NOT fatiguing the target muscles on your lead-up sets.

Nutrition

There is more to eating for muscle than just eating a lot of food. To truly maximize your muscle-building potential, you need to focus on quality, timing AND quantity.

These sections will take you through everything you need to know to get the most out of the *Mad Scientist Muscle* program. I will explain everything from caloric intake to sample recipes and recommended supplements.

I've also included a controversial addition to the program - low carb eating. This is an optional dietary technique you can use during specific days of the program that will help keep fat gain in check while at the same time hormonally prepping your body for enhanced muscle growth. It's definitely worth checking out!

IMPORTANT: Please keep in mind that I am not a medical doctor or nutritionist. This information is for educational purposes only and you should always consult your physician before making any major changes to your diet.

3 Simple Rules on Eating For Muscle Growth

Nutrition can be a very confusing topic. There's constantly new research coming out that says this nutrient is good, or this nutrient is bad, eat this, don't eat that, etc. It can be downright overwhelming.

And when things get overwhelming, the default response is to go back that with which you are most familiar. And if that wasn't getting you anywhere, then that's not a good thing.

So here it is, plain and simple. Nutrition for muscle growth is NOT complicated. I can break it into three basic rules for you.

1. Eat Plenty of Calories

Your body needs a caloric excess in order to most effectively build muscle. If you're not gaining muscle, there's a strong chance you're just not eating enough food. So if you've got training in order and you're still not gaining, eat more.

2. Eat Plenty of Protein

Aside from all the scientific arguments about how much we can digest and how much a person needs, there lies a simple truth: your body needs protein to build muscle.

If you don't eat enough, your body won't be able to build muscle effectively and that is definitely not what we're looking for. On the other hand, if you get too much, ABSOLUTELY NOTHING BAD HAPPENS (unless you've got kidney problems, but that's another issue).

You can debate the exact numbers all you want but none of it matters to your body if you don't eat ENOUGH.

3. Eat Good Quality Food and Drink a Lot of Water

This means stick to unprocessed, natural-state foods as much as possible (not necessarily low-fat, though). The more processed a food is, the more work your body has to do digest it, which takes energy away from the muscle-building process. It's a much bigger leap for your body to turn Corn Flakes into muscle than it is to turn a Sirloin steak into muscle.

So make it easy on yourself and stick to good food as much as possible, drink PLENTY of water and, while I'm at it, don't be afraid of vegetables either.

CONCLUSION:

There you have it! Muscle-building nutrition wrapped up into three simple rules. Follow them and you're on your way to massive muscle growth. These topics below will give you much more detailed information on actually implementing these three rules into your overall muscle-building program.

Caloric Intake	It's important to not only know what to eat, but how much of it to eat. Learn more about your optimal caloric intake for this program here.
Commonsense Protein FAQ	Here's the commonsense guide to protein intake for muscle-building... how much you need, how much your body can digest, can too much harm your kidneys, etc.

Meal Timing	WHEN you eat can be just as important as what and how much you eat. Learn the best way to time your meals around your training and how you can get great results on even just 3 meals a day!
The Low Carb Eating Option	How the heck could low-carb eating possibly fit in with a muscle-building program? I'll give you a hint...it can actually keep you LEAN while allowing you to build even MORE muscle.
Supplements	Here you will learn which supplements are useful and EXACTLY how to take them with this program to maximize your results.
Pre, Peri and Post-Workout Nutrition	Find out what you need to eat before, during and after a workout in order to take full advantage of both the training you're doing.
My "Lazy Cook" Muscle-Building Recipes	Preparing a good muscle-building meal doesn't have to be ridiculously hard and time-intensive. These sample meals are designed with the lazy cook in mind.
Eating Clean or Not Eating Clean?	Should you eat nothing but clean foods for best results, or is it actually GOOD to eat a little junk now and again, if your goal is maximum mass?

Caloric Intake

Though calorie-counting is not necessary on this diet, the number of calories you eat in a day is still important. No matter what kind of diet you're on, if you eat fewer calories than you burn, you will not gain very much muscle. You need to eat calories in excess of your maintenance level in order to gain mass.

The Basics of Caloric Intake

In order to gain muscle, you need to have a caloric surplus. What this basically means is that you need to take in more energy than you put out. For example, if your body needs 2000 calories per day to maintain its current weight, to increase your muscle mass, you'll need to eat MORE than 2000 calories per day.

The theory is simple but the execution can be confusing!

On the *Mad Scientist Muscle* dietary plan, we will be looking for a moderate to high caloric surplus of around **500 to 1000 calories above maintenance levels per day.**

The reason I give you such a wide range is that some people can gain quite well on just 500 or so extra calories a day and eating more than that would risk unnecessary fat gain.

On the other hand, some people do better with a greater caloric excess and actually NEED those extra calories to really make progress.

My recommendation is to start with the 500 and see how your results and energy levels are then increase as-needed from there.

The Bottom Line: In order to GET big, you have to EAT big, so don't be shy to eat substantial meals.

Maintenance Levels and Recommended Daily Caloric Intake Tables

If you ARE interested in counting calories, the following tables will give you a more specific idea of how many calories you should be eating per day while on this program. I will give general maintenance levels based on gender, age, weight and height as well as a range for daily caloric intake. We will assume a high activity level since you're doing this program.

Keep in mind, these are just general estimates and guidelines - not "set in stone" rules that you must follow! What your body requires may be far different than what's listed in a table or in a formula. When in doubt, go by your results. If you are not gaining muscle, it's safe to say you're eating too few calories. Adjust your intake higher at that point.

To find your numbers, find the weight that is closest to yours then the height that is closest to yours then the age that is closest to yours. The next row will tell you your approximate maintenance levels. The next row is your range of recommended daily caloric intake.

Note: these numbers have been calculated using the Harris-Benedict Formula for determining Basal Metabolic Rate (BMR). The BMR is the number of calories your body burns in a day just for keeping your body functioning. To get your maintenance level, we multiply that number (BMR) by a factor determined by your activity level. The higher your activity level, the higher your maintenance levels. The formula itself will be listed below the tables if you'd like to work with it yourself for your exact numbers.

Male:

Weight	Height	Age	Maintenance Level	Recommended Daily Intake
150 lbs / 68 kg	5' 0" / 152 cm	20	2520	3000-3500
		35	2362	2800-3300
		50	2204	2700-3200
	5' 6" / 168 cm	20	2639	3100-3600
		35	2480	2900-3400
		50	2322	2800-3300
	6' 0" / 183 cm	20	2757	3200-3700
		35	2599	3100-3600
		50	2440	2900-3400
170 lbs / 77 kg	5' 0" / 152 cm	20	2713	3200-3700
		35	2555	3100-3600
		50	2397	2900-3400
	5' 6" / 168 cm	20	2832	3300-3800
		35	2673	3200-3700
		50	2515	3000-3500
	6' 0" / 183 cm	20	2950	3500-4000
		35	2792	3300-3800
		50	2634	3100-3600
200 lbs / 91 kg	5' 0" / 152 cm	20	3003	3500-4000
		35	2845	3300-3800
		50	2687	3200-3700
	5' 6" / 168 cm	20	3121	3600-4100
		35	2963	3500-4000
		50	2805	3300-3800
	6' 0" / 183 cm	20	3239	3700-4200
		35	3081	3500-4000
		50	2923	3400-3900

Nick Nilsson

Female:

Weight	Height	Age	Maintenance Level	Recommended Daily Intake
150 lbs / 68 kg	5' 0" / 152 cm	20	2106	2600-3100
		35	1997	2500-3000
		50	1888	2400-2900
	5' 5 " / 165 cm	20	2142	2600-3100
		35	2033	2500-3000
		50	1923	2400-2900
	5' 10" / 178 cm	20	2177	2700-3200
		35	2068	2600-3100
		50	1959	2500-3000
145 lbs / 77 kg	5' 5 " / 165 cm	20	2311	2800-3300
		35	2202	2700-3200
		50	2092	2600-3100
	5' 10" / 178 cm	20	2346	2800-3300
		35	2237	2700-3200
		50	2128	2600-3100
170 lbs / 91 kg	5' 0" / 152 cm	20	2445	2900-3400
		35	2335	2800-3300
		50	2226	2700-3200
	5' 5 " / 165 cm	20	2480	3000-3500
		35	2371	2900-3400
		50	2261	2800-3300
	5' 10" / 178 cm	20	2515	3000-3500
		35	2406	2900-3400
		50	2297	2800-3300

The Harris-Benedict Formula

If you are interested in calculating your own specific numbers, here are the Harris-Benedict Formulas for men and women:

1 inch = 2.54 cm (multiply inches by 2.54 to get your height in cm)

1 kg = 2.2 lbs (divide your weight in pounds by 2.2 to get your weight in kg)

Mad Scientist Muscle

Men:

$66 + (13.7 \times \text{wt in kg}) + (5 \times \text{ht in cm}) - (6.8 \times \text{age in years}) = \text{BMR}$

Women:

$655 + (9.6 \times \text{wt in kg}) + (1.8 \times \text{ht in cm}) - (4.7 \times \text{age in years}) = \text{BMR}$

To find your maintenance levels, we must now multiply your BMR by your Activity Factor. I have used a factor of 1.55 in the tables above so as not to overestimate caloric requirements.

Sedentary	BMR x 1.2	Little or no exercise
Lightly Active	BMR x 1.375	Light exercise/sports 1-3 days/week
Moderately Active	BMR x 1.55	Moderate exercise/sports 3-5 days/week
Very Active	BMR x 1.725	Hard exercise/sports 6-7 days/week
Extremely Active	BMR x 1.9	Hard daily exercise/sports, and physical job, 2x per day training, marathon training, etc.

The resulting number will be your maintenance value. This is a general number and should only be taken as a guide, not as a rule. Add 300 to 500 calories to this number to get your daily caloric intake range.

Commonsense Protein FAQ

P rotein is the nutrient that is most commonly associated with weight training, yet it's also one of the most misunderstood. When it comes right down to it, when you train with weights, your body NEEDS protein.

But when it comes to using protein (both in supplement form and in food), there is a lot of confusion. In this FAQ, you're going to get common sense answers to some of the most frequently asked questions that people have about protein.

QUESTION #1: How Much Protein Does Your Body Really Need?

ANSWER:

At its simplest, your body has a baseline protein requirement that depends on a two main factors: lean body mass (muscle) and activity (type and amount).

The more muscle your body carries, the higher your protein requirement. Also, the more intense, the more frequent and the longer the activity you perform, the more protein you need.

Studies on protein requirements that demonstrate a greater need for protein often meet with much controversy in scientific literature. It seems sometimes, for some reason, that many in the scientific and nutritional community are actually anti-protein! In fact, you may have even witnessed a similar prejudice when it comes to supplements as simple as vitamins as well.

The Bottom Line: If you train with weights, your body is breaking down protein and you need to provide it with extra protein to help rebuild. Though the exact amounts that different sources recommend varies widely between 0.7 grams per pound of bodyweight (140 grams for a 200 lb person) to levels as high as 2 grams per pound of bodyweight (400 grams for a 200 lb person), there is a solution...

Experiment for yourself! Start with a moderate protein intake of 0.7 grams per pound of bodyweight and see how you feel and how your results are. The next week, increase your protein intake a little, adding about 20 to 30 grams to your daily total. See if that makes a difference. The following week, add a little more protein.

You may find that you need more protein than you've been taking or you may find that you don't need as much protein as you think.

My VERY general recommendation is to eat at least 1 gram per pound of boyweight - this will ensure you get plenty of protein.

On a side note, even when you read food labels and charts, EVERY piece of food you eat is different and every number you calculate is an estimate. Don't get caught up in the little things that don't make a difference. Get plenty of protein and don't stress yourself out worrying about it.

QUESTION #2: How Much Protein Can The Body Digest At One Time?

ANSWER:

There are many who suggest your body can't digest and use more than 30 to 40 grams of protein at a time. I've not seen convincing research on it to say if that's true or not.

Personally, using a common sense approach, I think we need to consider a few things.

1. Think about what state your body is in. If your body needs the protein (like after workout), I think it will use and digest more of it if it's available. Your entire metabolism is accelerated after a workout and protein use in the body shoots up. If protein is just eaten during the day, smaller servings of around 40 grams may well be better.

2. It's better to have more than you need than not enough when you need it. After a workout, I take in about 60 grams of whey protein, simply because, even if my body can't use it all, I'd prefer to have a little bit more than not have enough, which would slow down recovery.

 The same can certainly apply during the day. A little extra protein that your body burns up or excretes is not going to have any appreciable negative effects. But, not having protein available when your body needs it can slow and stop muscle growth.

3. Protein doesn't digest all at once, especially with meals. Think about it this way, your stomach doesn't process and send out everything it digests all at once. It works on some and then sends some on its way. This applies more to meals than protein drinks but the fact remains, your body doesn't digest a whole meal all at once. It digests a little at a time. Think of it like a time-release vitamin - your body doesn't use the whole thing all at once but uses it over the course of the entire digestion process.

Nick Nilsson

4. Different people can handle different doses of nutrients other than protein. Does it make sense that a 250 lb bodybuilder can only digest the same amount of protein as a 110 lb woman at one time? Different metabolic systems require and can handle different dosages.

The Bottom Line: The limit of 30 to 40 grams of protein at once could be right, but it could be wrong. Just make sure you're getting plenty if and when your body needs it.

QUESTION #3: Will Eating Too Much Protein Make You Fat?

ANSWER:

The quick answer to that question is yes. However, an excess of ANY nutrient (protein, carbs or fat) has the potential to make you fat. Of the three major nutrients, protein is the LEAST likely to do so as it's primarily a structural nutrient rather than an energy nutrient.

A common sense approach to answering this question would be to break it all down by numbers.

Consider this:

1 gram of protein contains 4 calories. Your body uses approximately 40% of the calories stored in protein to break it down and digest it.

Say you eat 300 grams of protein per day and your body only needs 150 grams. That's 150 extra grams of protein per day. Of those 150 grams (which yields 600 calories), the equivalent of 60 of those grams (240 calories) will be burned digesting the extra protein.

This leaves you with 360 extra calories. A pound of fat contains 3500 calories. It's going to take a LOT of excess protein to fill up a pound of fat. Even then, if you're training hard, excess calories are burned to fuel your activity (not necessarily from the protein itself but also from carbs and fat).

The Bottom Line: The fat-gaining effects of eating extra protein are negligible. You're better off making sure your body is getting enough protein when you're training hard.

QUESTION #4: Do I Need To Take Protein Supplements?

ANSWER:

The answer to this question is both yes and no.

You DON'T need to supplement with protein if you're getting enough quality protein in your food in your regular diet. You also don't need to supplement if you are able to get your protein conveniently and when your body needs it (especially after a workout).

If you can get enough protein and get it when your body needs it, there's no need to supplement with it. Food sources of protein are absolutely fine and you can build and support muscle with them.

But here's the big "BUT"!

Food sources are good for daily protein requirements BUT you SHOULD supplement with protein if you're not able to get enough quality protein in your diet WHEN your body needs it.

The very best example of this is after a hard workout. Protein supplements are easily digested by your body and very convenient to simply drink after a workout. This is the time when your body needs protein the most and getting it to your muscles quickly is a top priority. Food sources of protein are just not digested as quickly as supplements for post-workout use. Supplements are an easy way to make sure your body has the protein it needs after a workout.

Also, if you have trouble getting enough protein on a regular basis throughout the day, a protein supplement is ideal for keeping your muscles supplied consistently. It's much easier to drink a protein shake than cook and eat a chicken breast!

The Bottom Line: While you don't always HAVE to take a protein supplement, sometimes it's a very good idea. If nothing else, take a protein supplement IMMEDIATELY after a workout to maximize recovery and results.

QUESTION #5: Will Eating Too Much Protein Harm My Kidneys?

ANSWER:

No. It will only harm your kidneys if you already have trouble with your kidneys. No studies have demonstrated damage to the kidneys with increased protein intake unless the kidneys are already damaged.

Nick Nilsson

Drinking plenty of water can help the kidneys do their job of processing waste products, though! Keep in mind that there are many other variables at work in the body as well, including other bodily processes that could affect protein metabolism and excretion. If you have any concerns about protein and how your body uses it, I would definitely recommend you consult with your physician.

CONCLUSION:

These commonsense answers to frequently-asked protein questions should help you get a better idea of how you should look at and structure your protein consumption.

Meal Timing For Mass

One of the most frequent questions I get is about how often you need to eat to really get results. Much of the information you see tells you that you have to eat 5 or 6 meals a day in order to get good results. Well, here's the truth. You don't.

Oh, I'm not saying that you SHOULDN'T eat 6 meals a day and that it may not be better that way...I'm saying that it's not an absolute necessity and if you think you're screwed if you can't eat 6 times a day, get that thought out of your head.

In fact, you can eat THREE meals a day and do just fine with your muscle-building efforts. The key is your meal timing.

Like many people, sometimes job and family obligations mean that you can't always find the time to not only prepare but to even EAT 5 or 6 meals a day. But even if you can only fit in the standard 3 meals a day, you can still do just fine.

And many people simply find they can't eat big meals constantly throughout the day and find themselves just stuffed, which is not a good situation either.

If you choose foods that digest over a longer period and make sure you eat enough in your meals to keep yourself from getting too hungry, you're on the way.

Here's how I normally like to do it - I typically only get 3 or 4 meals a day myself (sometimes more if I count snacks).

Breakfast - Eat as soon after waking as possible. This should be a fairly big meal. I like to have something like oatmeal with yogurt in it for long-term energy with a big plate of scrambled eggs (don't be afraid to eat the yolks - that's where all the nutrients are and that's what makes eggs a complete protein - and forget the cholesterol in an egg...dietary cholesterol in the egg doesn't affect blood levels AND the egg yolk has enough lecithin in it to emulsify 3 times the amount of fat that is actually in the egg). This breakfast is enough to hold me until lunch time.

Lunch - This should be a somewhat lighter meal. This varies but it includes foods like protein shakes, tuna, peanut butter and jelly sandwiches, leftovers from supper the night before, fruit, veggies, salad, chicken breast, etc. The key that I like to go by here is to start with protein and eat that first. The reason for that (especially if you're working all afternoon) is that if you eat a carb-only lunch, your blood sugar will go up then back down and leave you sleeping at your desk. Protein keeps you awake and alert.

Training Afternoon/Early Evening - Enough hours have passed from lunch that I'm not training on a full stomach, which is ideal for growth hormone secretion. I don't like to have food in me when training. Take protein, simple sugary carbs and vitamins as a post-workout shake right after training.

Supper - About an hour after training, this should be your biggest meal of the day - you can take in upwards of 50% of your day's calories in your post-workout meal. Good source of protein, starchy carbs like potatoes or pasta or brown rice are fine after a workout - your body will use them. Try not to eat too late, especially if you go to bed fairly early. If I feel like it, I might take a protein shake before going to sleep - especially if dinner has digested fully. This should be a big enough meal that it doesn't leave you hungry for an unhealthy snack in the evening.

That's pretty much it!

This type of meal timing can really work well for those who have a hard time stuffing themselves with food constantly throughout the day. If you can commit to one BIG meal a day, you're all set.

Other Meal Timing Notes...

- You can work with your meal timing depending on when you train as well. If you train first thing in the morning, have a big breakfast after your training - don't skip that meal if you train in the morning. That'll leave you hungry all day or it'll slow your metabolism down and/or cause your body to cannibalize its own muscle tissue to help rebuild the damaged muscles.

- If you aim for those 3 meals then try and grab a healthy snack whenever you can, e.g. fruits, veggies, nuts, you'll get results.

- Your post-workout meal should be your BIGGEST meal of the day. This is when your body is primed for nutrient utilization. If you train early and that's breakfast, perfect. If you train in the evening and its supper, perfect, too! Just make sure you're getting a good load of calories in when your body is really going to make best use of them.

Even if it might be better to eat smaller more frequent meals, sometimes in the real world, it doesn't always work out that way. It's simple enough to go with the flow and get great muscle building results when you can at least control WHAT you eat, if not when.

The Low Carb Eating Option

If you've heard of the Atkins Diet, then you're probably familiar with low-carb eating. The premise of the low-carb diet (and there are many others besides the more-famous Atkins Diet) is simple: by depriving your body of its preferred fuel, the carbohydrate, you force it to rely on fat stores for energy.

So how in the heck does THAT fit in with a <u>MUSCLE-BUILDING</u> plan?

I'll tell you and it's for a number of reasons, all of which have the potential to force more muscle onto your body while keeping you lean.

And before I go any further, the low-carb/reduced-calorie eating is only going to be 2 days a week, IF you decide to give it a try. **It's totally optional** but I've found it to be an extremely useful technique for actually increasing muscle growth while keeping body fat gains to a minimum.

You can do it every week, every other week or even every third week - it's totally up to you. Here's why it works...

1. Carb Loading

When you restrict carbs, your body uses up its stores of glycogen (the form in which carbs are stored in your muscles and liver for later use by the body). Over the course of a day or two of restricted-carb eating, your body uses up all that stored glycogen.

Your body doesn't like being deprived...

So this deprivation sets up a need in your body to STORE as many carbs as it can when you introduce them back into your diet. You might be familiar with the term "carb loading" - that's exactly what this is all about.

When you go back to eating carbs, your body can store up to one and a half times the amount of glycogen as it normally would.

Now here's the thing - glycogen stores don't really do a whole lot for muscle growth directly BUT what happens when your body is rapidly taking up extra carbs into the muscles is that a lot of water and other nutrients (like amino acids) come along for the ride.

That is an EXTREMELY anabolic situation in your body. We're basically trying to mimic the effects of "rebound weight gain" that people on diets see when they come off a diet - only in a good way.

It's this anabolic inrush of nutrients and water that we're looking to take advantage of with the carb-deprivation and loading.

2. Insulin Sensitivity

One of the other big pieces of the puzzle with low-carb eating is insulin. Insulin is your body's primary storage hormone. It's absolutely <u>critical</u> for maximum muscle growth.

Here's an analogy to help explain how insulin works with muscle growth. Picture people going in the front door of a house one by one, they are getting inside the house but it's not particularly fast or efficient.

Your body CAN get amino acids and other nutrients into the muscles without high insulin levels, but when insulin levels are elevated, we open up the BIG garage doors and let a TON more people in at once. Insulin is the hormone that opens up the big doors and really lets the nutrients into the cells.

Granted, this can work on both muscle AND fat cells, so you don't want high insulin levels all the time.

You also want your body to be able to achieve that big-door effect with as little insulin as possible. The more sensitive your muscle cells are to the effects of insulin, the more bang for your buck you're going to get with insulin.

Here's the thing: When you eat carbs all the time, your insulin sensitivity decreases. You don't get the same big response as you do if you're more sensitive to it.

When you remove carbs from your diet, your body automatically begins to get more sensitive to the effects of insulin so when you do put the carbs back...BAM. The door opens and the carbs and other nutrients are able to come flooding in to the muscle cells.

3. Fat Loss

Low-carb eating is one of THE best ways to lose fat. It's a fact. By purposefully including very short fat-loss cycles into each week of the program, we're giving your body a chance to burn off any fat gains that might have happened over the previous 5 days.

After all, what good is to gain massive muscle if you just end up looking bigger and fatter? We want muscle without excessive fat gain.

These two days of lower-calorie, low-carb eating will accomplish exactly that. Because we're not doing any training on those low-carb days, muscle breakdown will be very minimal and won't be anything to worry about.

4. You Get To Eat More Fat

From a hormonal perspective, you need dietary fat in order to manufacture hormones such as testosterone. On the other hand, when you're looking to gain muscle without adding a lot of fat, you don't want to be eating tons of dietary fat, especially when insulin levels are high or it'll potentially get stored in the fat cells more easily.

So by increasing your fat intake on the low-carb days, you'll get the best of both worlds. You'll be able to take advantage of the hormonal benefits of higher-fat eating while keeping to somewhat lower-fat and higher-carb eating on the weekdays where you want higher insulin levels.

5. Resting the Digestive System

One of the biggest problems people have with gaining muscle is eating enough food to gain muscle.

The counterintuitive thing here is that simply trying harder to eat more and more food is NOT the best solution to that problem. All you're doing is stuffing more food into an already stuffed and overworked digestive system and that will get you nowhere.

By eating low-calorie and low-carb (which will basically be protein, healthy fats and veggies) for two days, you're going to help clean out your digestive system and give it a break from being stuffed full of food all the time. This will help it function more efficiently when you do go back to eating more again during the week.

The other benefit: eating less food for a few days is going to make you hungry! And there's nothing like being hungry to help increase your appetite.

How To Do Low-Carb Eating:

In order to eat a low-carb diet, you must reduce your carbohydrate intake to 30 to 50 grams per day. You can certainly go below this as well.

I normally recommend shooting for 30 grams a day as extra carbs have a way of sneaking into foods. Aiming for the low end means you'll be much more likely to stay within the proper range.

This is done by eliminating or drastically reducing intake of carbohydrate-containing foods such as breads, fruits, rice, pasta, cereals, grains, sugars, etc.

You will be focusing your food intake on low-carb foods such as meats, fish, poultry, healthy oils (fish oil, flax, hemp, borage, etc.), vegetables, salads and cheese.

It is essential that you read labels and know exactly what you're eating when you do low carb. There can be hidden carbs even in foods you may not think of as low carb.

To help you in the low-carb days of this program, I've provided resource links for more detailed information on how to do a low-carb diet. These sites explain in great detail how to follow a low-carb diet. On these sites, you'll find meal plans, charts of the number of carbs in certain foods, food to avoid, etc.

http://www.lowcarb.ca/

http://www.lowcarbluxury.com

http://www.lowcarbfriends.com/

http://atkins.com

My personal preference when eating low carb is to **focus primarily on natural, low carb foods such as meat, eggs, cheese, vegetables, salads, healthy oils, etc. rather than foods that are manufactured to be low carb.** This focus will definitely help you to keep your nutrition low carb.

To maximize the fat loss and health benefits of the low carb phase, you can also try eating fairly low-fat, low-carb foods while adding in healthy oils such as fish oil, flax oil, olive oil, etc. for energy.

I personally recommend **AGAINST eating bacon and sausage and other processed, fatty meats regularly** even on a low carb diet. They're okay as an occasional treat but don't rely on them as a regular part of your diet. Being on a low- carb diet should not be a license to eat garbage food, regardless of whether it is low carb or not. This food still needs to be processed by your body, after all!

Net Carbs, Effective Carbs and Impact Carbs - Good or Bad?

While keeping track of net carbs, effective carbs and impact carbs may be good for some, I personally don't recommend frequently eating foods that rely on these definitions and alterations. Naturally low carb foods, in my opinion, are simply better for you.

The less processing a food has been through, the easier it is for your body to work with. Manufactured low-carb foods are, in many cases, just the same junk food repackaged in a low-carb format to give the appearance of "healthy." **My recommendation is to eliminate or minimize the use of these foods.** The body simply wasn't designed to digest the large amounts of sugar alcohol that most of these rely on to sweeten their products.

Low-Calorie Eating:

In addition to eating low-carb, we also want to be relatively low-calorie, with a moderate caloric deficit of about 300 to 500 calories per day.

You can figure out your maintenance levels using the formula on the Caloric Intake page.

In addition to the hormonal and carb-loading effects of these two days, the reduced calorie levels will also set up a deficit and a physical need in your body to catch up.

We really want to take full advantage of rebound weight gain here!

With these two days, if you don't want to try low-carb eating, it might be worth trying out at least low-calorie eating. It won't give you quite the same rebound as low-carb but it will definitely rest the digestive system and give you a moderate rebound.

"Cheat" Meal:

Since you're already eating a fair bit of food during the week and not really dieting strictly, it might be a bit of a stretch to call this a cheat meal...but I'm going to anyway.

This meal should be eaten as your post-workout meal after the Friday training session. We want this to be a BIG meal. Eat foods you might not normally eat even on a regular muscle-building diet. The idea here is to spike your metabolism right before you hit two days of low-carb eating.

Muscle-Building Supplementation

Supplementation can really help maximize your results on the *Mad Scientist Muscle* Program. We will be using basic supplements - you don't need anything fancy. How you use them and when is what really gets you the results! I will go through what to use, exactly when to use it and why.

Please note, I am not a nutritionist or doctor and you should always consult with your health professional before adding any supplements into your diet. This page is presented for informational purposes only. My supplement recommendations are all very safe for the general healthy population but I don't know your exact situation.

1. Multivitamins

First on the list are multivitamins. Food simply does not have enough nutrients in it these days to allow even the healthiest eater to get optimal amounts of vitamins and minerals, even when eating regular meals and even when eating a surplus of calories. Think of a multivitamin as an insurance policy. It helps to protect you from any deficiencies you could get and not even know about.

- Don't take generic, low-quality multivitamins. You may as well be swallowing little rocks for all the nutrients you will get out of them.

- Most vitamins (including popular brand names) that come in tablet form are so compressed that they can't be broken down even by stomach acid.

- Look for multivitamins in capsule or gelcap form. These will be the most absorbable.

When To Take It:

A multivitamin should be taken on EVERY day of the program. If your multivitamin serving calls for multiple doses, you can separate them over the course of the day for optimum absorption, e.g. morning and evening.

2. Protein

Protein is the building block of muscle tissue. Without enough protein, all your training efforts will be for naught because your body won't have the raw materials to recover and rebuild.

Protein is readily available in food, true, but protein-containing foods are not always the most convenient to prepare or eat. When was the last time you packed some scrambled eggs into your backpack for a snack?

When To Take Protein:

Protein can and should be taken during every day of the program. It's not so critical on non-training days, since protein turnover will be lower, but it can definitely help with overall growth and recovery.

Here is a list of the when, why and how of effective protein supplementation, ranked in order of importance.

1. Immediately After A Workout

If you only take protein once per day, this is the absolute best time to take it. Immediately after you finish your workout, your body needs raw materials to rebuild and recover with. If you don't supply the raw materials through eating, your body will break down muscle from elsewhere in your body in order to rebuild the damaged areas. This is very counterproductive as you can well imagine.

By taking in some protein (20 to 40 grams or so, depending on bodyweight - take 0.2 g/lb of bodyweight) within minutes after exercise, you provide your body with the raw materials it needs to recover without breaking down its own muscle tissue.

2. Immediate Before A Workout

Right before you train, taking in a small amount of protein can help turn in-workout catabolism into anabolism. A small 10 gram dose of protein along with a 30 to 35 gram dose of sugar can promote better growth and recovery - its well worth taking.

3. First Thing In The Morning

Immediately upon waking, or as soon after that as you can manage, take a scoop of protein powder. Your body has just been through an 8+ hour fast and is hungry for nutrients. Feed your body!

Protein powder is more quickly assimilated than solid food and gets into your muscles faster. This protein shot gives your metabolism a boost, which can help with fat loss. Be sure to follow it with a good breakfast, of course.

4. Last Thing At Night

Prepare your body for the long overnight fast by giving it a little something to work with. A good combination for this purpose is to mix a scoop of whey protein in with a small glass of milk.

Whey is what's known as a "fast" protein, meaning that it's digested quickly, while milk protein (casein) is what's known as a "slow" protein, meaning it's digested relatively slowly. At night, you want your protein to be metabolized slowly so that your body gets a more even supply over the course of the night. By mixing "fast" and "slow" proteins, you get the benefits of the higher-quality whey with the slower digestion time of the milk.

5. In-between Meals

A quick protein shake can be a great snack in between meals. It helps keep your body supplied with protein all day long. This is especially useful if you tend to have long periods of time in-between meals. It could mean the difference between losing muscle and building or keeping muscle.

6. With Meals

Taking a protein supplement with meals is a handy way to increase the protein content of a meal. This is perfect for when you make a meal that is somewhat low in protein.

7. In The Middle Of The Night

This is a trick that bodybuilders sometimes use in order to keep their muscles supplied with protein throughout the night. Keep a premixed protein shake right beside your bed. Although some trainers have been known to set alarms to wake up to drink it, don't do that. Just have it there waiting just in case you wake up, but don't try to wake up on purpose - you're better off getting good, solid sleep. If you don't wake up during the night, its right there ready to drink first thing in the morning!

3. Joint Supplements

Next on the list is a good joint supplement. Here's the deal...you can't train nearly as heavy when your joints are sore. When you train heavy (and if you don't take joint supplements), your joints WILL get sore.

I consider joint supplements to be **<u>ESSENTIAL</u>** supplements for any serious trainer, even before creatine. Your joints have to last you a lifetime. You take care of them and they'll take care of you!

So you MUST take a good joint supplement. You simply cannot get enough joint support nutrients through diet alone. Your body needs raw materials to repair and rebuild the joints and if you don't provide it through diet, your joints will eventually get ground down.

This is especially true when you're doing partial training (which is a big part of the Structural phase) that is directly targeting the connective tissue. When you break down muscle tissue, you provide protein to help it rebuild. The same goes for joints and connective tissue - if you target them, you MUST support them nutritionally.

Here's a list of the best joint support nutrients:

> **Glucosamine** 1500 mg per day (500 mg taken 3 times a day is good)
>
> **Chondroitin** 400 to 600 mg per day **MSM** 1 to 2 grams per day
>
> **Hyaluronic Acid** follow label instructions **Vitamin C** 1000 to 5000 mg per day
>
> **Gelatin** 1 to 5 grams per day (varies) **Calcium** 1000 to 1500 mg per day

4. "Greens" Supplements

The reality is that probably 99% of us don't get enough veggies in our diets. I shouldn't have to repeat that this is a huge problem, but I do, both to readers and clients. So unless you're getting 6 servings of fruits and veggies per day, greens products should make up the difference.

These "greens" products contain powdered concentrates of a huge variety of healthy fruits, vegetables and other plants, giving you a nice spectrum of a variety of nutrients.

You can pick up "greens" supplements at most health food stores. Greens+ is an excellent brand. I've also used Barley Green in the past, with excellent results and stores like Trader Joes and Whole Foods will have their own store brands as well.

When To Take It:

A "greens" supplement can and should be taken on every single day of the program. It's nutritional insurance that can really make a difference in your results and your health.

5. Fish Oil/Essential Fatty Acids

Essential Fatty Acids are so-named because it's essential to get some in your diet. Without them, your health and body composition will suffer. Unfortunately the typical North American diet is low in Linoleic Acid (an omega 6 fat) and in Alpha Linolenic Acid (an omega 3 fat); therefore we typically have to seek additional supplementation.

Furthermore, even if the EFA content of the diet seems acceptable, the all-important ratio of omega 3 fats to omega 6 fats is often askew, with far too much omega 6 and far too few omega 3s.

While the omega 3 fat Alpha Linolenic Acid is important in the diet, the downstream metabolic products of ALA (DHA and EPA) are powerful fats responsible for things like: increased metabolic rate, improved fat burning, increased carbohydrate storage in muscle, better glucose and insulin tolerance, reduced blood lipids, reduced risk of platelet aggregation, cardiovascular disease, cancer, and diabetes.

To get your DHA and EPA, you've got to go with fish oil or krill oil. There are lots of fish oils and krill oils on the market to choose from and manufacturers make it confusing to decide which is best. Quality makes a HUGE difference with fish oil and krill oil, though, so I definitely don't recommend the cheap Sam's Club bulk bin types of fish oil.

EFA's are EXCELLENT anti-inflammatories and with the heavy training you're doing on this program that can make a HUGE difference in how you feel after your workout sessions. This is a highly recommended supplement.

When To Take It:

You should take EFA's on every single day of the program. This is a supplement that is constantly useful.

I like to recommend people "load up" on fish oil supplements, taking about 6 to 10 grams a day for the first week, in order to saturate their body with the EFA's. After that, you can back to half or less of that for a maintenance dose, in order to maintain levels in your body.

6. Creatine Monohydrate

Creatine Monohydrate is an excellent muscle-building supplement. It is completely safe to use for both men and women. There are many scientific studies documenting its safety and effectiveness. It is a natural substance found primarily in red meat.

Using creatine can cause a rapid weight gain of approximately 3 to 10 pounds during the loading phase, depending on the amount of muscle and water you are carrying right now. The bigger you are, the more weight you will gain. This weight is primarily in the form of more water in your muscles.

Creatine builds strength by increasing the amount of fuel available for muscle contractions. By increasing your available fuel, your body is able to lift more weight and do more reps. This, in turn, allows you to build muscle.

When To Take It:

Creatine users typically load up for a period of 5 days then drop down to a maintenance dose to keep high levels in the muscles. I recommend staying on this maintenance dose for about 4 to 6 weeks, then coming off creatine for at least 2 to 3 weeks.

Take 5 grams of creatine four times a day for the first 5 days of the program then scale back to a single 5 gram dose for the rest of the days, taken before or after training.

On non-training days, take your creatine any time in between meals.

When loading, I like to take a dose first thing in the morning, an hour before training and immediately after training. The final does is taken any time in between meals.

I personally take regular, plain creatine monohydrate. I get excellent results with the no-frills version. There are a number of supplements on the market that claim to take creatine supplementation to the next level. My suggestion is to try regular creatine the first time through so you have a basis to compare to. Then try the fancier stuff. If you find you get enough results to justify the higher cost, go for it!

7. Glutamine

Glutamine is a nonessential amino acid in the body but it is also the most abundant amino acid in the body. Around 50% of the free amino acid pool consists of glutamine.

Taking extra glutamine has a variety of beneficial effects on your body.

- A dosage of 2 grams on an empty stomach has been shown to increase the level of circulating Growth Hormone in the body. This is good because Growth Hormone promotes muscle growth and fat loss, which are the major aims of this program.

- Another effect is that the body does not have to break down other amino acids to make glutamine. Glutamine is a popular amino in the body and if glutamine levels are low, the body will break down muscle protein to synthesize it.

- The extra glutamine you take in supplement form helps support muscle growth if taken in doses of 5 grams or more at a time (this large amount is necessary to get enough past the digestive system to be of value - the gut sucks up glutamine like a sponge).

- Other effects of glutamine include immune system boosting, improved recovery, cell volumization and enhancement of glycogen replenishment.

The best times to take glutamine are first thing in the morning, right after a workout and right before sleep.

- Dosages can vary from 2 grams (minimum) to about 10 to 15 grams or more. The larger doses should be used immediately after a workout to promote anabolism and minimize catabolism (muscle breakdown).

When To Take It:

Glutamine should be taken after every workout. It will help your body recover quickly from the intense training you are putting yourself through. It will also help keep your immune system functioning at peak levels as you push yourself towards overtraining over the course of the program. This is a critical time - if your immune system is down, you'll be more likely to get sick at this time.

Also, glutamine works in a similar fashion to creatine by carrying water into the muscle cells as it gets absorbed. This cell volumizing effect dramatically enhances muscle cell growth.

A side benefit to taking plenty of glutamine is the positive effects it has on strengthening the immune systems, especially as you get near the end of the Accumulation Phase where your training volume has increased a lot. Your body will be pushed to the edge and this will tend to reduce immune system functioning. Glutamine can help keep you from getting sick during this time. It's very effective!

Glutamine is easiest to take in powder form. Capsules are available but you need to take so many of them to get a decent effect, it's not really worth it. Regular glutamine powder should work perfectly.

8. Leucine and Branch-Chain Amino Acids

Leucine is a critical amino acid when it comes to muscle growth. By taking supplemental Leucine, you can immediately "turn on" anabolism.

Adding Leucine to your protein drinks and/or your food is an easy way to really punch up the muscle-building power of your diet.

Branch-Chain Amino Acids (leucine, isoleucine and valine) can be taken to achieve a very similar effect. You can get them in capsules, powder and even liquid form.

When To Take It:

Leucine and/or BCAA's can be taken before and during workouts to help flip the switch to anabolism. Leucine powder can also be taken with meals in order to improve the anabolic capabilities of that meal. This can be especially useful when eating a relatively low-protein meal.

These are excellent between meals, especially if you find you'll be going a longer time without being able to get anything to eat.

9. Vitamin D3

Vitamin D isn't going to directly help you build muscle - I'll tell you that right up front. What it WILL do is help keep you from getting sick while you're accumulating volume and moving towards overtraining.

When you hit that level of overtraining, your body becomes rundown and more susceptible to illness. Your immunity is lower and we've got to take that into account! That last thing you want to happen is to get halfway through the program then get sick right when you're about to hit the most productive phase of the program!

You can get Vitamin D through sun exposure on your skin but most people simply don't get enough through this and many people are critically deficient. Sunscreen will prevent the factors in your skin that create Vitamin D and if you shower or bathe within 24 hours of sun exposure, it washes off those factors as well!

Getting Vitamin D via dairy products is ok, but that form is not well absorbed, which is why the recommendation for supplement D3.

When To Take It:

Vitamin D3 is the most bio-available form of Vitamin D and can be taken any time throughout the day. Take at least 1000 IU's - there have been no documented toxicity cases at this range and recommendations from health professionals can be 2000 to 4000 IU's a day, depending on body levels. Starting with 1000 IU's should be fine.

10. Other Vitamins and Minerals

I'll tell you right now, there is nothing glamorous about taking minerals and vitamins. You will NEVER see a full-page ad in

Muscle & Fitness for the latest calcium supplement or see Mr. Olympia plugging a B vitamin complex.

But simple, basic nutrients like minerals and vitamins are absolutely CRITICAL for EVERYBODY who trains with weights. I'm going to give you a few of the major ones you need to be aware of and be sure you're getting enough of them. A full discussion of all the major minerals and vitamins you need is well beyond the scope of this book but the ones I'm going to mention can make a BIG difference in your training and FAST.

You can get pretty much any of these things at any health food store, GNC or local drugstores and grocery stores. I prefer to buy online and eliminate the middleman. It keeps prices down quite a lot.

1. Calcium

Calcium makes up the majority of the mineral weight in your body (your bones). It's VERY important to take supplemental calcium - your body simply doesn't absorb it well from most foods. You may drink a lot of milk, but not much of that calcium is actually getting absorbed by your body.

Ideally, you should take in about 1000 mg to 1500 mg of calcium per day. This will support bone health and a host of other processes that calcium is required for (including blood clotting, nerve function and muscle contraction). Without enough calcium, you will be compromising your long-term health. If you don't provide enough in your diet, your body will PULL IT OUT OF YOUR BONES to get it.

Calcium excretion is actually INCREASED when you're eating a high-protein diet, making it doubly important for those looking to increase muscle mass to get plenty of calcium.

Vitamin D is required for optimal calcium absorption, so look for that in any calcium supplements you purchase. Be sure that you don't go above 2000 mg per day in calcium supplementation. Also, calcium intake should be balanced with magnesium intake (I'll talk more on this below). The ratio should be 2 to 1 calcium to magnesium, which would be 1000 mg calcium to 500 mg magnesium.

The best sources (in terms of absorbability) of supplemental calcium are calcium citrate and calcium citrate malate. Coral calcium is also purported to be a highly absorbable form of calcium. Many calcium products also include magnesium in them.

2. Magnesium

Magnesium is one THE most important minerals in the body. It is essential for a multitude of processes (more than 300) yet is often missing completely from both food and supplementation regimens. While true magnesium deficiency is rare, you can benefit greatly from getting optimal levels of it. Magnesium is critical for cellular energy production as well as the structure of your body (bones especially) and the healing process.

Bottom line, if you're not getting enough magnesium, your strength will suffer. When you start getting optimal levels, you will probably notice a strength increase fairly rapidly.

Magnesium intake should ideally be balanced with calcium intake (the 2 to 1 ratio I mentioned above). The range of 300 to 400 mg per day is considered a minimum intake for healthy adults (depending on bodyweight). You can take an additional 300 to 400 mg per day supplemental. The easiest way to tell if you're taking too much supplemental magnesium…let's just say, larger doses of magnesium have a laxative effect...

The easiest way to go with magnesium is to just purchase it in a formula combined with Calcium. That way, you can just take one pill instead of doubling up. The citrate form of magnesium is one of the better absorbed versions.

3. Zinc

Zinc is another critical mineral in the body that, like magnesium, is required for many of the chemical reactions and processes in your body. Zinc acts as a catalyst in many of these reactions. Zinc also plays a critical role in the structure of proteins and cell membranes as well as being important for immune system function and anabolic hormone production (e.g. testosterone).

Most multivitamins have some level of zinc in them but you may benefit from taking a 25 mg to 50 mg zinc supplement on its own. DO NOT go above 150 mg per day for more than a few days. Zinc is one mineral where it is possible to get adverse reactions at a relatively low dose. More is NOT better in this case.

4. Vitamin C

Vitamin C is another totally unglamorous supplement that can have tremendous effects on your training and health and is a MUST HAVE. The amount necessary to stave off deficiency is about 60 mg per day. The amount for optimal health and performance is MUCH greater than that, especially when you're training your muscles hard and working on connective tissue as major goal.

Vitamin C is an essential component in the synthesis of collagen, which basically is what connective tissue is made of!

Without enough Vitamin C, collagen formation will grind down. For our purposes in this program, we want to ensure we're getting PLENTY of Vitamin C. Personally, I take about 3,000 to 5,000 mg per day of it. The good part about Vitamin C is that it's water-soluble. This means excess levels are easily and quickly flushed out of the body.

One of the other important functions of Vitamin C is as an antioxidant. It's very effective at quashing free radicals, which is a BIG concern when training hard. To prevent cell damage, antioxidant intake is vital.

Also, we can't forget the effects of Vitamin C supplementation on cortisol levels. Cortisol is the stress hormone associated with stress and muscle breakdown. Three 1000 mg doses of Vitamin C during the day can decrease cortisol levels very effectively, which will help a LOT with staying anabolic. Think you're a hard gainer? Maybe you're not getting enough Vitamin C.

Lastly, **Vitamin C taken before a workout (500 mg to 1000 mg) can actually help reduce muscle soreness**, which is VERY useful on this program, especially on the Structural weeks of the program.

You can take pretty much any version of Vitamin C - there hasn't been research proving any one form is any better than any other form.

11. Pre and Post Workout Supplements

Pre-workout and post-workout supplementation can make a BIG difference in your recovery and your results. Good pre- workout nutrition can give your body a supply of nutrients to prevent the catabolic state that you normally get into during training. Post-workout nutrition helps with faster recovery.

Ironically enough, research has demonstrated that the ratios of carbs to protein in pre and post-workout feedings should be the SAME for optimum results.

A Summary of How To Take All These Supplements

Having all these supplements is one thing - taking all of them properly is another. Here's a quick guide to help you get it right.

1. Multivitamin	Ideally, you want to take this in divided doses 2 or 3 times a day, e.g. morning, post- workout and last thing at night.
2. Protein	Post-workout, first thing in the morning, with meals, between meals.
3. Joint Supplements	Take 2 or 3 times a day, e.g. morning, post-workout, last thing at night.
4. Creatine	Load up at the start of the program and stay on it all the way through the full cycle on a maintenance dose.
5. Glutamine	Take 10 to 20 grams after every workout. On non-training days, you can take it just before bed.
6. Calcium & Magnesium	Take 2 or 3 times a day in divided doses, e.g. morning, post-workout and night.
7. Zinc	Just once later in evening (can take with other vitamins last thing at night)
8. Vitamin C	Take 3 times a day in divided doses (1000 mg each time). Also 500 to 1000 mg 45 minutes before training.
9. Fish Oil	Take 2 or 3 times a day in divided doses (1 to 3 grams each dose)
10. Vitamin D3	This can be taken twice a day, with your other vitamins.

11. Leucine and BCAA's	Leucine can be taken with meals to improve the anabolic quality of the meal. It can also be taken in between meals, as can BCAA's (which are also effective before and during training).
12. "Greens" Powder	You can take this anytime. I usually take it mixed in with protein powder in the morning and evening or post-workout.
13. Pre/Post Workout Formula	Self-explanatory.

Naturally, you don't NEED to take ALL of these supplements to get results with the program. **I would at the very least suggest a good multivitamin and a joint support supplement. These are the basics, in my opinion.**

Once you've got your basics taken care of, you can start try some "exotic" supplements to see how they work for you and add to your results.

In the end, you'll get better results from your training and nutrition if you focus your supplementation on SUPPORTING the process rather than on having supplements trying to BE the driving force behind your results. Supplements won't lift that heavy barbell for you and lifting that heavy barbell is what REALLY drives your results forward.

Pre, Peri and Post- Workout Nutrition

Pre-Workout Nutrition

How you perform in your training sessions is going to be determined a fair bit by what you eat in the time leading up to it. In general, if have plenty of protein and good quality calories, you'll perform just fine.

How about <u>RIGHT BEFORE</u> your training sessions, though? What should you eat (or should you eat at all?) before you train in order to perform at your best during the workout?

A study done on this exact question has shown that taking in a combination of simple carbs and protein in a ratio of approximately 5 to 1 (carbs to essential amino acids) immediately before exercise can shift the body from catabolism (muscle breakdown) during a workout to anabolism (muscle-building).

The study was done using a fairly small dose - 35 grams of sucrose and 6 grams of essential amino acids (aminos that your body must take in because it can't manufacture them itself - 6 g works out to about 10 grams of a "complete" protein source like whey) and the results actually showed a greater positive effect on muscle anabolism than the same formula taken AFTER training.

So this pre-workout nutrition is definitely important stuff!

What I would recommend would be a half scoop of vanilla whey protein (which is generally about 20 grams of protein, so a half scoop would be 10 grams) mixed with about 35 grams of a sugary drink mix like Tang. There are supplements specifically designed for pre-workout but, to be honest, a lot of them are just filled with extra stuff you don't need that hasn't been proven to do anything for muscle growth (e.g. Nitric Oxide).

Ironically enough, taking in TOO MUCH protein in pre-and post workout shakes can actually set you back by actually reducing insulin secretion by causing the insulin-antagonist hormone glucagon to be secreted. Make sure you don't overload on protein either before or after - it's the insulin release along with the presence of a decent amount of protein that will do the trick for you.

Branched-Chain Amino Acids can be an excellent choice for your pre-and post workout supplementation, especially Leucine. Research has also shown that just taking BCAA's gives you comparable anabolic effects to complete proteins.

If you don't want to use supplements, even something as simple as a glass of chocolate milk will get the job done (as long as you're not lactose intolerant!).

Remember, if you find you do better when you don't take anything before training, that's fine. It's not going to totally make or break your results if you don't take a pre-workout supplement.

It CAN give you a muscle-building boost, but if you can't do it, don't worry about it!

Peri-Workout Nutrition

Peri-workout nutrition, in this case, means what you take in DURING your workout. Sipping a similar drink to what you took in pre-workout can continue to help fuel the muscles while training.

Personally, I prefer to just drink water while training. If you're taking a pre-workout supplement, you'll pretty much have your bases well covered so I don't feel the need to recommend taking something during training.

Post-Workout Nutrition

When you exercise, your body burns fats and carbohydrates for energy and breaks down your muscle tissue. Immediately after a workout, the body has an enhanced ability to utilize nutrients such as glucose and protein in order to rebuild and recover from your exercise.

What this essentially means is that your body is turbocharged and ready to grow! This period of power lasts for approximately four hours after a workout, hence the name "**Four-Hour Window of Opportunity.**"

Taking in nutrients immediately after exercise helps you to recover faster and feel better after a workout. This can help you gain muscle faster AND keep your metabolism fueled so that you lose fat at a faster rate.

But what happens if you don't eat immediately following a workout? Let me put it this way: it's definitely a situation you want to avoid.

First, your body starts breaking down muscle tissue in undamaged areas of your body in order to get raw materials to help repair the areas you just worked. Over time, this will result in a loss of muscle from your whole body.

Stress hormones in the body (primarily a hormone called cortisol) speed this process along. The stress hormones are produced because working out is a stress on the body - it's a totally natural but results-stopping reaction. How do you control the effects of cortisol? You eat as soon as you can.

But what do you eat after a workout to maximize your results? Both protein and carbohydrates are important for fast recovery.

* Protein

Immediately following a workout (within a few minutes of completion) take some protein. The easiest and best way to do this is in the form of a protein powder (whey is an excellent choice and is digested quickly). Although, a food source such as milk works if you don't have any supplement options.

Taking protein gives your body something to rebuild with instead of tearing down its own muscle tissue for raw materials. Try to get at least 20 to 40 grams of protein in as soon as you can after you're done (the amount depends on your bodyweight).

Take in 0.4g/kg bodyweight (which works out to about 0.2g/lb) of protein hydrolysate, e.g. whey protein.

So if you weigh 220 lbs/10 kg, you would take in about 40 to 45 grams of whey protein post-workout. If you weight 150 lbs/68 kg, you would take in about 27 to 30 grams of whey protein.

* Carbohydrates

Take in about 40 to 80 grams of simple carbohydrates to help the body refuel (depending on bodyweight). Your body is most efficient at rebuilding its carbohydrate stores immediately after a workout. It's important to take advantage of this period.

Right after a workout is one of the few times where simple carbs (sugary, quick to digest carbs) are actually very useful. The simple carbs will help your body to make use of the other nutrients you are putting in by raising insulin levels in the body. The insulin helps to shuttle these nutrients into the muscle cells.

Simple carb intake should be about double your protein intake post-workout. This works out to 0.8g/kg of bodyweight (0.4 g/lb). It's a pretty straightforward two to one ratio of carbs to protein to maximize insulin response and amino acid uptake into the muscle cells.

* Fats

It is important to minimize your fat intake following your workouts. Post-workout fat intake has been shown decrease circulating Growth Hormone levels to HALF [Reference #10]. Naturally, this is not something we want to happen. That being said, a small dose of healthy fats, such as flax oil, can have positive effects on recovery.

Post-Workout Meal

About one hour after your workout, take in a high quality source of protein (as in the examples above) and a good supply of carbohydrates such as grains, potatoes, cereals, etc. At this time, the body has settled down from the stress of the workout and is looking to rebuild.

If you're looking to get as much from your workouts as you possibly can, you can see that post-workout nutrition is critical. By supplying an ample amount of raw materials right after you're done, you will be preventing the body from breaking itself down in order to recover. This means more results from the effort you put into your workouts!

Do You Count Post-Workout Supplements in Your Daily Calories?

That's a very common question. In my experience, it's not necessary to include post-workout supplements in your daily calorie totals, assuming you're not going TOO nuts with the protein and carbs.

So bottom line, don't count those calories towards your daily totals.

My "Lazy Cook" Muscle- Building Recipes

If you're like me, you sometimes find yourself short on time to cook yourself a good meal. And if you're also like me, meaning a lazy cook, sometimes the motivation to really make a grand meal is short, too!

So what do you do when this happens but you still want to reach your muscle-building goals?

I've got three great "recipes" (and I use the word "recipes" in the loosest sense possible) to share with you that will help you stay on track towards massing up.

Keep in mind that even though I'm going to inject a little humor into this list, these are examples of actual things you can prepare for yourself to help make your life easier. I just want to show you that decent nutrition doesn't have to be dull as dirt or taste like it either.

> **It's important to note, I'm NOT a nutritionist and I don't claim to be!** So PLEASE don't make a gigantic vat of mashed potatoes then complain because you're diabetic and your blood sugar is so high that you're sweating maple syrup. These recipes are for "entertainment purposes only," so if you DO follow them **personal responsibility** is the keyword here! :)

These recipes are simple to make, don't take long to cook and are geared to my own personal skill level of cooking, which is pretty basic

1. Spaghetti with Cajun Meat Sauce

This is a great, protein-rich post-workout meal. Tastes great and serves 1 to 4 people, depending completely on how hungry you are and your willingness to share with others.

- 1 pound of whole wheat spaghetti

- 1 jar of sauce that's thick enough to cover up the taste of whole wheat spaghetti (that's my own opinion, at least!)

- 1 pound of lean ground beef (I like ground sirloin for this because it's leaner)

- Some prepackaged Cajun spices - I get big containers of these at Sam's Club but most grocery stores should have some version. This really spices up the meat sauce nicely.

First, put some water in a big pot and set the stove on high to bring it to a boil. Fill a sauce pan/fry pan about halfway up with water. I like to put the ground beef in the pan BEFORE I add the water so it doesn't splash all over the place when I dump in the meat (I found THAT out the hard way, of course - the dog was happy about the meat water all over the floor but the shirt I was wearing will never be the same).

Bring the water in that pan to a boil and throw a bunch of Cajun spice in the pan with the meat. Don't be cheap with it! Stir it in and smash the meat up so it's not all clumped together.

Once the spaghetti water is boiling you can dump in the spaghetti. Let it boil for 9-10 minutes then drain. The meat will be boiling while the spaghetti is boiling - if the meat gets done first, drain it then cover it up. It'll keep its heat as long as it's covered.

Empty the sauce jar into the spaghetti pot and stir it up. If you're not sharing the pasta with someone who doesn't like meat, feel free to throw the meat in the spaghetti pot, too. If you ARE sharing, serve out some spaghetti into a separate big bowl THEN toss the meat in there. It'll just work out better for all concerned that way.

Serve sitting on the couch with an oven mitt under the bowl because it'll be hot on the bottom! And it's better NOT to wear a white shirt while you're eating it. 'Nuff said.

2. Scrambled Eggs and Oatmeal With Yogurt And Fruit

This is a great breakfast meal that will keep you from getting hungry for HOURS. The fat in the egg yolks keeps you satisfied while the thick oatmeal will keep your digestive system busy for a long time. Lots of fiber to work on!

- 6 whole eggs - not egg whites, WHOLE eggs! They're not bad for you like many people seem to think. The yolk is where most of the nutrients are — they taste a whole lot better with yolks, too. Adjust the number of eggs to your preference.

- 1 gob of Smart Balance margarine to coat the bottom of the pan. Cooking spray will work for this as will olive oil.

- 1 dry cup of Quaker Oats - either the Old Fashioned or 1 Minute oats are fine. Adjust the quantity of oats to your preference.

- 2 cups of water (basically, double the amount of oats you put in).

- A bunch of fruit - whatever your favorite fruit is. I find berries or grapes work best because you don't need to cut them up. Wash them before eating them.

- 1 Thing of yogurt - this is the technical term for however much yogurt you want to put in the oatmeal. If I have individually packaged yogurts, I'll just dump one of those in. If I have a bigger container, I'll scoop a pile of yogurt in until it looks like enough. You'll figure out how much you want to put in.

First, get the fruit ready. Wash it up and put it in a small bowl. Crack the eggs into a bowl/cup and scramble them. If you're talented, you can crack them with one hand and not slop them down the sides. After cracking about 30,000 eggs in my lifetime, I'm still not talented. I managed to do it once then the next time I ended up with a dripping fistful of egg and shell.

** On a side note, it IS possible to squeeze an egg with one hand and break it. A friend of mine once told me that you can't put an egg in the palm of your hand, squeeze it and break it. He said it wasn't possible (he was a physics major). So I grabbed an egg and squeezed it REALLY tight. Three seconds later, it exploded so hard the yolk popped out and flew 6 feet across the room and actually landed right in his shirt pocket!

Anyway, THAT being said, measure out a cup of oats, dump it in a good-sized bowl, then add double the amount of oats in water, e.g. 1 cup of oats, add 2 cups of water. You can adjust the water later, depending on if you like your oatmeal a little soupy (like I do) or masonry thick (like my wife does).

Nuke it in the microwave for about 3 minutes or boil it on the stove in a pot, both work. While that's going, turn on the stove and get the pan for the eggs heated up. Throw a gob of Smart Balance margarine in the pan (that's a great brand - it's actually a reasonably healthy margarine and tastes good). Olive oil and nonstick spray will do the trick, too. With the olive oil, it's a good idea to have a spray bottle for it so it doesn't all pool up in the corner that your stove burner leans to (you know what I'm talking about).

Make sure the whole bottom surface of the egg pan gets covered with something slippery or you'll regret it later when you try to keep eggs from getting all crusted up and nasty along the sides.

Pour the beaten eggs into the pan and watch them cook. Stir them around once the bottom starts to get solid. Keep stirring and scraping the sides off to avoid the crust I mentioned above.

Your oatmeal should be done about the same time the eggs are. So put the eggs on a plate and set it aside for now.

Take your bowl of oatmeal then dump the yogurt in, then the fruit. Stir it all up (not the eggs, just the fruit and yogurt) and you're good to go.

This meal will keep you going for hours!

3. Meat and Taters

"Meat and potatoes" might be a cliché but for me, there's not much that works better for supporting muscle growth than a nice piece of meat (or chicken or fish) and a big bucket of potatoes. And if that sounds corny, it should, because sometimes I'll throw some corn in with the potatoes.

Let's talk about potatoes first, then I'll give you the inside scoop on how to cook meat (I think I can hear my wife laughing in the background as I write about my cooking skills...).

First, grab 3 or 4 good-sized potatoes. I try to get red potatoes since they can't be stored as long as other potatoes therefore they're fresher when you get them rather than having been sitting in storage for a year.

I like to microwave potatoes since it's faster than boiling and they turn out really well but boiling works really well, too.

Wash any crud off them then slice off any questionable areas. Stick a fork or knife in them a few times to "aerate" so they don't explode in the microwave (unless you enjoy scraping your dinner off the sides).

For each potato, figure on about 3 to 5 minutes of cooking time, depending on the size of your potato and power of your microwave. You'll know they're done when you can easily stick a fork right through - just don't leave the fork in the microwave or you'll be in for a surprise.

If you boil the potatoes instead, cut them up into smaller chunks so they cook faster. If you just throw in whole potatoes, you'll be in for a bit of a wait. When sliced up, they'll take about 20 minutes or so at a full boil.

Dump them in a big bowl, mix in some margarine (or if you're on a low-fat kick, pour some ketchup in it), add some sea salt and you're set. You can also throw in a can of corn (nuke it or boil it first - not the can but the corn) to spice things up.

As for the meat, if you're good with a gas or charcoal grill - more power to you. You're a better cook than I am and I don't know why you're even reading this part.

If you have one of those George Foreman countertop grills, those work really well for meat (especially the ones that you can pull the grill things off and put them in the dishwasher). Follow the instructions that came with the grill for the meat or chicken or fish you're cooking.

If you've got some chicken breasts that you just want to "fire and forget" rather than tend to on a grill, throw them in pan, preheat the oven to about 400 degrees, dump some spices on them (whatever you like), cover with tinfoil to keep the juices in, and cook for about 30 minutes or so (SET THE TIMER!). If you want to get REALLY fancy, slice up a lemon and toss a few slices on top with some black pepper.

There you have it. Meat and potatoes. Perfect for a big post-workout meal that will help you pack on the pounds.

I also like to use potatoes, corn and ground beef (or sirloin) to make "Lazy Cook" Shepherd's Pie. Microwave the potatoes and corn as above. Boil the meat as in recipe #1, then dump it all into a big bowl and stir. You'll be 5 pounds heavier by the end of the meal!

Conclusion:

As you can see, cooking tasty food for building muscle doesn't have to be hard and recipes don't have to be these complex things that take hours to make and require more than very basic cooking skills. With my recipes, if you can do a few simple things without burning yourself, that's about all the skill you need.

Eating Clean or
Not Eating Clean?

This is one of the big questions people have about eating for muscle growth...should I eat clean and try and get enough calories from healthy foods or should I eat some "junk" foods in order to consume more easy calories.

The definition of eating "clean" is basically sticking with unprocessed, natural-state foods that are relatively low in fat. For example, clean would be chicken breast and brown rice with salad. "Not clean" would be along the lines of hamburgers, pizza, French fries and other foods that are processed to varying degrees.

And the answer to the question of eating clean or not is...it depends.

It depends on several things...

1. Are you able to get enough calories and protein eating clean?

If you ARE, then you'll have no problem gaining muscle on a clean diet. In my experience, I've found some people seem to actually thrive on the occasional "junk" food thrown in because of the influx of fats, carbs and other nutrients (and yep, grease counts as a nutrient...not a good one, but it is a fat, nevertheless!)

Plus, one of the nice things about being on a weight-gain diet is you do have the ability to be a bit more "free" with your eating, which makes social get-togethers easier to manage (easier than having everybody look at you strange when you order a boiled chicken breast at a restaurant, anyway!). I don't look at it as a license to go nuts, but having a little more leeway in your eating can be a good thing.

2. Are you very concerned about gaining some extra fat with your muscle?

If you ARE very concerned about adding extra fat, then the choice is clear: eat clean as much as possible and do your best to get enough calories. Increase your good fats, such as olive oil, in order to add calories to your diet. Get plenty of lean protein and don't be afraid of egg yolks (they're actually really quite good for you!).

My Real-World Solution:

My philosophy is one that includes BOTH. Eat the majority of your meals "clean," especially when you're at home and can easily control what you eat. When you do eat "not clean" meals, it's best to do so purposefully rather than by accident and have those as a post-workout meal so your body has the best chance of making use of all the extra calories and fat, etc. rather than storing it.

In the program itself, if you're doing the "Low Carb Option," I also like to purposefully include a "cheat" meal on Friday (post- workout) because I'll be going right into low-carb dieting the next day.

The bottom line: Try and eat the majority of your meals clean, but if you need the extra calories, sometimes a big pizza is just what the doctor ordered. Just don't make a habit of it.

A Note About Alcohol Use:

Alcohol use should be eliminated or greatly minimized while you are on the *Mad Scientist Muscle* program. Alcohol is known for its detrimental effects on both fat-burning and muscle-building hormones and its use can severely hamper your results. Save your alcohol use for when you're not on the program, if you want the best results possible on the program.

APPENDIX
The Mad Scientist Muscle Programs

Here are the THREE 8-week training programs (that's six months of training) for you to use and experiment with. These will keep you getting great results and keep your training FUN for a LONG time!

You can do these training cycles in ANY order, so if any one cycle appeals to you more, you're free to start with that. Each one can stand alone on its own.

Miscellaneous Program Notes

1. Detailed Training Program Charts

For each program's 8 week cycle I've included a general overview and then a more detailed day-by-day breakdown.

Each Training Day is placed in a very specific order of what to eat and how to train. Follow the instructions as closely as possible to get the best results possible.

These programs are constructed as a numbered day system, not for specific days of the week, though the programs are designed around "weekday" training.

2. Cardio and Sports Practices

Cardio training is never done on the same day as a weight training session, unless it's low-intensity, such as walking or other easy exercise. I have included some optional cardio training sessions in the program with cardiovascular-maintenance as the goal, not necessarily fat loss. This cardio is in the form of aerobic interval training.

The reason cardio is optional in the program is that some people simply do not grow well when extra calories get devoted to cardio training. The weight training you'll be doing will definitely work your cardiovascular system, though (especially during the accumulation phases where you're reducing rest periods), so even if you do ZERO cardio, you're not going to have issues in that department.

If you participate in a sport and have practices, try to separate your practices from your weight training sessions as much as possible so that you're not compromising your recovery from the weights and slowing down your gains.

3. The Low-Carb Option

Throughout the entire 8 weeks of each cycle of the program, I'm giving you what I call the "Low-Carb Option." What that means is, instead of eating "normal, high-calorie" the whole way through, you can do low-carb eating on the two days of the weekend.

It's TOTALLY optional, though, so don't freak out if you can't or don't want to do it, but definitely read more about the rationale behind it. It really does have the potential to not only enhance your muscle gains but to minimize fat gains that often come with the eating of excess calories during a muscle-building program.

You can also choose to do it SOMETIMES...meaning you can try it once and if you don't like it, no worries. You can do it every other week. You can do it every third week - it's an option and it's completely up to YOU.

What I like about the Low-Carb Option is that it takes the measuring and guesswork out of your eating, if you want to make sure you're gaining minimal body fat while you build muscle. You don't have to think about quantities - just eat low-carb on the weekends and the rest takes care of itself.

4. Changing up the Training Days for Greater Recovery

These cycles are set up according to a weekday-training schedule, meaning all the weight training is done during the week. This would be a Monday, Tuesday, Thursday, Friday schedule.

For greater recovery and training "fresher", you can adjust this so that you move the Friday session to Saturday (e.g. Monday, Tuesday Thursday, Saturday).

This gives you another day of rest between the last two sessions of the week - it can help with recovery, allowing you another day of being relatively rested when you go into a training session. If you can only train during the week, the original schedule will work just fine, though

If you decide to go this route AND you want to the Low-Carb Option, just do ONE day of low-carb eating on Sunday, even on the Intensification weeks. The Compound Exercise Overload training is extremely tough on the nervous system and doing only one day of low-carb will help with recovery.

Cycle 1 ~ Time/Volume Training

Week 1 - Structural

Week 2 - Volume - Time/Volume

Week 3 - Volume - Time/Volume

Week 4 - Volume - Time/Volume

Week 5 - Structural

Week 6 - Intensity - Low-Rep Strength Training

Week 7 - Intensity - Low-Rep Strength Training

Week 8 - OFF/Deload/Fun/Strength Test

Week 1
Structural Training

Day 1	Day 2	Day 3	Day 4	Day 5	Day 6 & 7
High-Rep Moderate Weight High-Speed Stretch sets	100's Stretch sets		Heavy Partial Training or High-Rep Partial Training	Heavy Partial Training or High- Rep Partial Training	
Back Chest Thighs Shoulders Hamstrings Biceps Triceps Calves	Chest Back Thighs Shoulders Hamstrings Biceps Triceps Calves	Rest	Chest Back Biceps Hamstrings	Triceps Shoulders Thighs Calves	Rest Cardio option

Weeks 2, 3, 4 -
Volume Time/Volume Training

You will follow the same basic program outline for all three weeks here, increasing your workload by increasing the number of sets you do with the shorter rest periods and increasing the weight as you're able to.

Day 1	Day 2	Day 3	Day 4	Day 5	Day 6 & 7
Chest Back Biceps Triceps	Thighs Shoulders Hamstrings Calves Abs	Rest	Chest Back Biceps Triceps	Thighs Shoulders Hamstrings Calves Abs	Rest

Week 5
Structural Training

Day 1	Day 2	Day 3	Day 4	Day 5	Day 6 & 7
High-Rep Moderate Weight High-Speed Stretch sets	100's Stretch sets		Heavy Partial Training or High- Rep Partial Training	Heavy Partial Training or High- Rep Partial Training	
Back Chest Thighs Shoulders Hamstrings Biceps Triceps Calves	Chest Back Thighs Shoulders Hamstrings Biceps Triceps Calves	Rest	Chest Back Biceps Hamstrings	Triceps Shoulders Thighs Calves	Rest Cardio option

Weeks 6 and 7 - Intensity
Low-Rep Strength Training

You will follow the same outline for both weeks of the Low-Rep Strength Training part of the program, using the same exercises and rep and set structure to provide a training effect so your body knows what to adapt to. Every body part will be worked with 3 sets (5-3-1 reps).

Day 1	Day 2	Day 3	Day 4	Day 5	Day 6 & 7
Chest Back Biceps Triceps	Thighs Shoulders Hamstrings Calves Abs	Rest	Chest Back Biceps Triceps	Thighs Shoulders Hamstrings Calves Abs	Rest Cardio Option

Week 8 - OFF/Deload/ Fun/Strength Test

Day 1	Day 2	Day 3	Day 4	Day 5	Day 6 & 7
Rest	Rest	Fun!	Rest	Strength Test 1 RM's	Rest Cardio option

Body part	Exercise	Sets	Reps	Notes
Back	Deadlifts, Row or Chin/Pulldown	1	20+	The preferred exercise is the deadlift. If you select a row, the 1 arm dumbbell; row or cable row beats barbell rows.
	Stiff-Arm Pushdowns or Dumbbell; Pullovers	1	4-6	These exercises focus on the overhead stretched position of the lats.
Chest	Any Barbell or Dumbbell; Bench Press Variation	1	20+	Don't bounce the bar off your chest as you lower it down. As well, don't bang the dumbbell;s together at the top.
	Any Dumbbell; Fly Variation	1	4-6	I like to use a Swiss ball fly for this as I find it gets the best stretch at the bottom and allows you to wrap your back around the ball.
Thighs	Barbell Squats, Dumbbell; Split Squats, Leg Press, Goblet Squat	1	20+	Squats will be hardest. The split squats lets you push until you can't stand up. With the Leg Press you can push without having to balance.
	Sissy Squats	1	4-6	If you can't do sissy squats because of knee issues, substitute just a plain quad stretch here instead.
Delts	Barbell or Dumbbell; Shoulder Press or Hang Clean & Press	1	20+	Use a lighter weight than you think you'll need for this - you'll be doing this after all the big body parts.
	W Presses or Leaning or Cable Laterals	1	4-6	There aren't many stretch exercises for shoulders - do your best to get a stretch with any of these.
Hams	Leg Curls	1	20+	These are going to burn. The hamstrings aren't well suited to high rep training.
	Stiff-Legged Deadlifts	1	4-6	Raise your toes onto a couple of weight plates to increase the stretch on the hams at the bottom.

Biceps	Barbell, Dumbbell; or	1	20+	Try to minimize body momentum when doing these - there will be a tendency to swing.
	Preacher Curls Incline Dumbbell; Curls	1	4-6	Sit up higher on the incline bench so your feet are on the seat and your upper back is off the top of the bench. You'll get a better stretch on the biceps.
Triceps	Close Grip Bench (decline or flat), Dips, Bench Dips, Pushdowns	1	20+	I like decline bench for close grip pressing. Pushdowns are a good option, if your shoulders and chest are fatigued.
	Overhead Ext. or Bodyweight Extension	1	4-6	Bodyweight extensions are excellent here - you can adjust the stretch and resistance on the fly.
Calves	Standing or Seated Calf Raises	1	20+	Either will work. You can actually do both parts of this on the same apparatus - just increase the weight for the stretch part.
	Donkey Calf Raises or Standing Calf Raises	1	4-6	Donkey calf raises will give you a better stretch.
	Core Combo	4	-	2 sets of abs - 1 set of lower back - 1 set rotator cuff

General Comments:

- Choose a weight that allows you to hit at least 20 reps. You'll want to do these FAST and explosively! Remember, you're doing just ONE set of the exercise so make it count.

- You'll get 20 seconds of rest then you'll do a stretch-focused exercise for that same body part. Hold the stretch for at least a 5 count on every rep. The idea here is to fill the muscles with blood on the first set then stretch the fascia on the second set.

- Take 90 seconds rest in between body parts.

Your Written Notes:

_____

_____

_____

_____

Mad Scientist Muscle - Day 2 - Structural Training

Body part	Exercise	Sets	Reps	Notes
Back	Row or any Pulldown Variation	1	100	No deadlifts here. A pulldown or rowing movement is good - use a two arm version so you don't have to switch back and forth between arms.
	Stiff-Arm Pushdowns or Dumbbell Pullovers	1	4-6	These exercises focus on the overhead stretched position of the lats.
Chest	Any Barbell or Dumbbell Bench Press Variation	1	100	Don't bounce the bar off your chest as you lower it down. Don't bang the dumbbells together at the top.
	Any Dumbbell Flye Variation	1	4-6	I like to use a Swiss ball flye for this as I find it gets the best stretch at the bottom and allows you to wrap your back around the ball.
Thighs	Barbell Squats or Leg Press or Leg Extensions	1	100	Leg press is the best choice here as it requires no stablization. Squats are going to be tough - yo may I need short rest periods.
	Sissy Squats	1	4-6	If you can't do sissy squats because of knee issues, substitute just a plain quad stretch here instead.
Delts	Barbell or Dumbbell Shoulder Press	1	100	Keep an eye on form on these - it will tend to break down fast when you hit the limit.
	W Presses or Leaning or Cable Laterals	1	4-6	There aren't many stretch exercises for shoulders - do your best to get a stretch with any of these.
Hams	Leg Curls	1	100	These are going to burn...the hamstrings aren't well suited to high rep training.
	Stiff-Legged Deadlifts	1	4-6	Raise your toes onto a couple of weight plates to increase the stretch on the hams at the bottom.

Biceps	Barbell, Dumbbell or Preacher Curls	1	100	Try to minimize body momentum when doing these - there will be a tendency to swing.
	Incline Dumbbell Curls	1	4-6	Sit up higher on the incline bench so your feet are on the seat and your upper back is off the top of the bench. You'll get a better stretch on the biceps.
Triceps	Pushdowns, Close Grip Bench (decline or flat), Dips	1	100	I prefer to use the decline bench for close grip pressing. Pushdowns are a good choice for this as they will isolate the triceps well.
	Lying Extensions, Overhead Ext. or Bodyweight Extensions	1	4-6	Bodyweight extensions are excellent here as they allow you to adjust the stretch and resistance on the fly.
Calves	Standing or Seated Calf Raises	1	100	Either will work
	Donkey Calf Raises or Standing Calf Raises	1	4-6	Donkey calf raises will give you a better stretch.
	Core Combo	4	-	2 sets of abs - 1 set of lower back - 1 set rotator cuff

General Comments:

- Use different exercises than you used on Day 1

- Choose a light weight that will target you for 100 reps...it will be tough to gauge this exactly but this first workout allow you to set some benchmarks so you know what to expect in future rounds through.

- If you can't get 100 reps, then do as many as you can...take 10 seconds rest then do as many more as you can. Continue till you get to 100 total.

- You'll then get 20 seconds rest then you'll do a stretch-focused exercise for that same body part. Hold the stretch for at least a 5 count on every rep. The idea here is to fill the muscles with blood on the first set then stretch the fascia on the second set.

- Take 90 seconds rest in between body parts..

Your Written Notes:

_____

_____

Mad Scientist Muscle - Day 3 - Rest

Body part	Exercise	Sets	Reps	Notes
None				

General Comments:

- This is a day of rest.

Your Written Notes:

_____

_____

Mad Scientist Muscle - Day 4 - Partial Training

Body part	Exercise	Sets	Reps	Notes
Chest	Barbell Bench Press	4	4-6	Just the top few inches on the bench press movement.
Back	Deadlifts	4	4-6	Also known as rack pulls. Make sure you're not using your thighs to leverage the weight up. Start the lift with the bar set just above the knees.
Hamstrings	Stiff-Legged Deadlifts or Leg Curls	3	4-6	The SLDL is the preferred exercise here. Use leg curls only if you absolutely can't do SLDL's. You can keep the same rail setting in the rack when you come right from the deadlifts.
Biceps	Barbell Curls	3	4-6	Keep your core VERY tight with this.
	Core Combo	7	-	3 sets of abs - 2 sets of lower back - 2 sets rotator cuff

General Comments:

- If you don't have a power rack, go with high-rep partial training instead. It'll be safer than doing heavy partials without a rack.

- For high-rep partials, you'll still use a fairly heavy weight but do partial reps in the strongest range of motion for very high reps (30 to 40+)

- Take at least 90 seconds rest in between sets.

- Try and hold the lockout positions for a 5 count in order to fully load the bones and connective tissue.

Your Written Notes:

_____

_____

_____

Mad Scientist Muscle - Day 5 - Partial Training

Body part	Exercise	Sets	Reps	Notes
Triceps	Decline or Flat Close Grip Bench or Weighted Dips	3	4-6	Close Grip Bench is the best one to use here. You can also use Weighted Dips, hitting only the top range of motion.
Shoulders	Barbell Military Press or Seated Dumbbell Press	3	4-6	The Barbell Shoulder Press is the best option for partial training. Dumbbells should only be used when you can't do barbells for this.
Thighs/ Quads	Squats or Leg Press	4	4-6	Lockout Partial Squats are BY FAR the best exercise to use here. Only use leg press if you absolutely can't do partial squats.
Calves	Standing Calf Raises	3	4-6	You can actually use the same power rack set up for partial calf raises as you did for squats, if you want to do barbell calf raises just in the top half of the range.
	Core Combo	7	-	3 sets of abs - 2 sets of lower back - 2 sets rotator cuff

General Comments:

- If you don't have a power rack, go with high-rep partial training instead. It'll be safer than doing heavy partials without a rack.

- For high-rep partials, you'll still use a fairly heavy weight but do partial reps in the strongest range of motion for very high reps (30 to 40+)

- Take at least 90 seconds rest in between sets.

Your Written Notes:

_____

_____

_____

Nick Nilsson

Mad Scientist Muscle - Day 6 & 7 - Rest

Body part	Exercise	Sets	Reps	Notes
None				

Cardiovascular Training	
Activity	**Comments**
Aerobic Interval Training	This is an OPTIONAL cardio training session done on Day 6 <u>ONLY</u>. Go for 15 to 20 minutes using any of the work to rest intervals listed on the Aerobic Interval Training page, e.g. 2 minutes work to 30 seconds rest intervals. The idea here is not to push yourself hard but to just maintain cardio capacity.

General Comments:

- The cardio training for this day is optional. If you find that doing cardio slows down muscle growth, you can opt not to do it.
- From a nutritional standpoint, treat your cardio session as a regular training session and have a post-workout meal and supplementation.

Your Written Notes:

_____

_____

_____

Mad Scientist Muscle - Day 1 - Time/Volume Training

Body part	Exercise	Time	Reps per Set	Notes
Back	Deadlifts, Chin-Ups, Barbell Rows or One-Arm Dumbbell Rows	15min	3	Deadlifts are the preferred exercise here since they involve the most muscle mass.
Chest	Barbell Bench Press or Dumbbell Bench Press	15min	3	Barbells are easier to work with - all you have to do is re-rack the weight after each set. With dumbbells, you have to set them down then pull them right back up into position again. It can be done but it'll drain you a bit more.
Biceps	Barbell, Preacher or Dumbbell Curls	7.5min	3	Any of theses exercises is fine here.
Triceps	Dips (weighted), Decline or Flat Close Grip Bench Press, Lying Tricep Extensions	7.5min	3	I prefer to use Decline Close Grip Bench Press or Weighted Dips for this session in order to maximize the weight load on the triceps.
	Core Combo	4	-	2 sets of abs - 1 set of lower back - 1 set rotator cuff

General Comments:

- You will be using the Time/Volume Training style today. You will be doing 3 rep sets for a designed time period. Select a weight you could normally get about 10 reps with.

- Stay strict with your 10 seconds in between mini-sets when you start. When you can no longer get 3 reps, increase rest to 20 seconds...then 30 seconds...then 40 seconds, as needed.

- Do not push to failure on any sets.

- If you can make it past 1/3 of the time without having to go to 20 seconds rest, then you'll increase the weight on that exercise in the next workout.

Your Written Notes:

_____

_____

_____

Mad Scientist Muscle - Day 2 - Time/Volume Training

Body part	Exercise	Time	Reps per Set	Notes
Thighs	Barbell Front Squats or Dumbbell Split Squats	15min	3	The best exercise to use here is the Front Squat, especially if you did deadlifts on the previous day. If you're using split squats, take your rest period in between legs, e.g. left then 10 sec rest, right then 10 sec rest, etc.
Shoulders	Seated Dumbbell Press or Barbell Military Press	7.5min	3	The Barbell Press will generally be easier to manage as you won't have to get the dumbbells up into position on every set. Dumbbells still work just fine, though (use a Preacher Curl bench facing backwards, if you have one).
Hamstrings	Stiff-Legged Deadlifts or Leg Curls	7.5min	3	SLDLs are the preferred exercise here. Leg curls are ok, but the deadlifts will hit a lot more muscle mass and really challenge you.
Calves	Standing, Seated, Donkey or Leg Press Calf Raises	7.5min	5	Any calf exercise will work equally as well here. The leg press calf raise will be the easiest to get into position. We're aiming for 5 rep sets for calves, since they generally respond better to a bit higher rep ranges.
	Core Combo	4	-	2 sets of abs - 1 set of lower back - 1 set rotator cuff

General Comments:

- You will be using the Time/Volume Training style today. You will be doing 3 rep sets for a designed time period. Select a weight you could normally get about 10 reps with.
- Stay strict with your 10 seconds in between mini-sets when you start. When you can no longer get 3 reps, increase rest to 20 seconds...then 30 seconds...then 40 seconds, as needed.
- Do not push to failure on any sets.
- If you can make it past 1/3 of the time without having to go to 20 seconds rest, then you'll increase the weight on that exercise in the next workout.

Your Written Notes:

_____

_____

Mad Scientist Muscle - Day 3 - Rest

Body part	Exercise	Sets	Reps	Notes
None				

Cardiovascular Training	
Activity	Comment

General Comments:

Your Written Notes:

_____

_____

_____

Nick Nilsson

Mad Scientist Muscle - Day 4 - Rest

Body part	Exercise	Time	Reps per Set	Notes
Back	Deadlifts, Chin-Ups, Barbell Rows or One- Arm Dumbbell; Rows	15min	3	If you used deadifts on Day 1 of T/V training, choose a different back exercise here, e.g. rows or chins/pulldowns.
Chest	Incline Barbell Bench Press or Dumbbell; Bench Press	15min	3	If you did flat bench on Day 1, use an incline version here..
Biceps	Barbell, Preacher or Dumbbell; Curls	7.5min	3	Any of theses exercises are fine here.
Triceps	Dips (weighted), Decline or Flat Close Grip Bench Press, Lying Tricep Extensions	7.5min	3	I prefer to use Decline Close Grip Bench Press or Weighted Dips for this session in order to maximize the weight load on the triceps. Use a different exercise than you did on Day 1
	Core Combo	4	-	2 sets of abs - 1 set of lower back - 1 set rotator cuff

General Comments:

- You will be using the Time/Volume Training style today. You will be doing 3 rep sets for a designed time period. Select a weight you could normally get about 10 reps with.

- Stay strict with your 10 seconds in between mini-sets when you start. When you can no longer get 3 reps, increase your rest to 20 seconds...then 30 seconds...then 40 seconds, as needed.

- Do not push to failure on any sets.

- If you can make it past 1/3 of the time without having to go to 20 seconds rest, then you'll increase the weight on that exercise in the next workout.

Your Written Notes:

_____

_____

_____

Mad Scientist Muscle - Day 5 - Time/Volume Training

Body part	Exercise	Time	Reps per Set	Notes
Thighs	Barbell Squats or Dumbbell Split Squats	15min	3	The best exercise to use here is the Barbell Squat - it'll involve the most muscle mass and really push you hard.
Shoulders	Seated Dumbbell Press, Barbell Military Press, or Hang Clean and Press	7.5min	3	The Hang Clean and Press is a good one to try here, if you've used it before. It'll hit the traps as well as the shoulders.
Hamstrings	Stiff-Legged Deadlifts or Leg Curls	7.5min	3	If you used SLDL's on Day 2, go with Leg Curls here. If you're advanced and comfortable with the exercise, you can also try Good Mornings.
Calves	Standing, Seated, Donkey or Leg Press Calf Raises	7.5min	5	Any calf exercise will work equally as well here. The leg press calf raise will be the easiest to get into position. We're aiming for 5 rep sets for calves, since they generally respond better to a bit higher rep ranges.
	Core Combo	4	-	2 sets of abs - 1 set of lower back - 1 set rotator cuff

General Comments:

- You will be using the Time/Volume Training style today. You will be doing 3 rep sets for a designed time period. Select a weight you could normally get about 10 reps with.

- Stay strict with your 10 seconds in between mini-sets when you start. When you can no longer get 3 reps, increase rest to 20 seconds...then 30 seconds...then 40 seconds.

- Do not push to failure on any sets.

- If you can make it past 1/3 of the time without having to go to 20 seconds rest, then you'll increase the weight on that exercise in the next workout.

- Since you're doing abs as part of the Time/Volume Training, no need to include them in the Core Combo

Your Written Notes:

_____

_____

_____

Nick Nilsson

Mad Scientist Muscle - Day 6 and 7 - Rest

Body part	Exercise	Sets	Reps	Notes
None				

Cardiovascular Training	
Activity	**Comment**
Aerobic Interval Training	This is an OPTIONAL cardio training session done on Day 6 <u>ONLY.</u> Go for 15 to 20 minutes using any of the work to rest intervals listed on the Aerobic Interval Training page, e.g. 2 minutes work to 30 seconds rest intervals. The idea here is not to push yourself hard but to just maintain cardio capacity.

General Comments:

• The cardio training for this day is optional. If you find that doing cardio slows down muscle growth, you can opt not to do it.

• From a nutritional standpoint, treat your cardio session as a regular training session and have a post-workout meal and supplementation.

Your Written Notes:

_____

_____

_____

Mad Scientist Muscle - Day 1 - Low Rep Strength Training

Body part	Exercise	Sets	Reps	Notes
Chest	Flat Barbell Bench Press or Dumbbell Press	3	5-3-1	Don't let your elbows flare out as you lower the weight. Be sure to keep your shoulder blades tight in behind your back.
Back	Deadlifts	3	5-3-1	Don't let your lower back round over when performing deadlifts.
Biceps	Barbell Curls	3	5-3-1	Keep your knees slightly bent and keep your entire body tight. A loose body will lead to cheating reps.
Triceps	Close Grip Bench Press (flat or decline) or Weighted Dipss	3	5-3-1	Decline close grip bench will allow you to load more weight onto the triceps.
	Core Combo	4	-	2 sets of abs - 1 set of lower back - 1 set rotator cuff

General Comments:

- You'll be doing 3 sets for each body part...5 reps on the first set, 3 reps on the second set and 1 rep on the third set. Increase the weight on each set, unless you don't hit the target reps.

- Take 90 seconds to 2 minutes rest between each set.

- Don't push to failure on any sets. Always keep the do-or-die rep in you.

Your Written Notes:

_____

_____

_____

_____

_____

Nick Nilsson

Mad Scientist Muscle - Day 2 - Low Rep Strength Training

Body part	Exercise	Sets	Reps	Notes
Thighs	Front Squats	3	5-3-1	Front squats will build up your core in addition to hitting the quads hard.
Shoulders	Military Press or Hang Clean and Press	3	5-3-1	The hang clean and press is a great "power" exercise. It also hits the traps really well.
Hamstrings	Stiff-Legged Deadlifts	3	5-3-1	To focus even more on the hamstrings, set your forefoot area
Calves	Standing or Seated Calf Raises	3	5-3-1	Hold the top and bottom positions of the calf raise for at least 2 to 3 seconds to maximize the effect.
Traps	Barbell or Dumbbell Shrugs	3	5-3-1	Use a powerful, explosive movement for shrugs.
	Core Combo	4	-	2 sets of abs - 1 set of lower back - 1 set rotator cuff

General Comments:

- You'll be doing 3 sets for each body part...5 reps on the first set, 3 reps on the second set and 1 rep on the third set. Increase the weight on each set, unless you don't hit the target reps.
- Take 90 seconds to 2 minutes rest between each set.
- Don't push to failure on any sets. Always keep the do-or-die rep in you.

Your Written Notes:

_____

_____

_____

_____

_____

Mad Scientist Muscle - Day 3 - Rest

Body part	Exercise	Sets	Reps	Notes
None				

Cardiovascular Training	
Activity	Comment

General Comments:

Your Written Notes:

_____

_____

_____

Nick Nilsson

Mad Scientist Muscle - Day 4 - Low Rep Strength Training

Body part	Exercise	Sets	Reps	Notes
Chest	Incline/Decline Barbell Bench Press or Dumbbell Press	3	5-3-1	If you used flat barbell bench on the first day, go with Incline or Decline press here, if you still want to use barbells. You can also use dumbbells for the chest on this day, too. The Swiss ball works well for those.
Back	Weighted Chin-Ups, One Arm Dumbbell Rows or Barbell Rows	3	5-3-1	Weighted chins or One Arm DB Rows are great for this. Use the DB rows before you do BB rows, if you have a choice. You'll be able to focus more effort onto one side of the body at a time and use relatively more weight.
Biceps	Dumbbell Curls	3	5-3-1	Do these alternating one arm a time, not both arms at the same time. It'll keep your form better and allow you to focus more neural drive onto one arm, making you a bit stronger.
Triceps	Close Grip Bench Press (flat or decline), Weighted Dips or Lying Tricep Extensions	3	5-3-1	Use whichever exercise you didn't use on Day 1 for triceps here. Weighted dips are a good option - just be careful of your shoulders and don't bounce at any point in the movement.
	Core Combo	4	-	2 sets of abs - 1 set of lower back - 1 set rotator cuff

General Comments:

- You'll be doing 3 sets for each body part...5 reps on the first set, 3 reps on the second set and 1 rep on the third set. Increase the weight on each set, unless you don't hit the target reps.

- Take 90 seconds to 2 minutes rest between each set.

- Don't push to failure on any sets. Always keep the do-or-die rep in you.

Your Written Notes:

_____

_____

_____

Mad Scientist Muscle - Day 5 - Low Rep Strength Training

Body part	Exercise	Sets	Reps	Notes
Thighs	Barbell Squats	3	5-3-1	If you can't do regular squats, use leg presses or dumbbell split squats.
Shoulders	Seated Dumbbell Shoulder Presses	3	5-3-1	Use strict form on these - don't overload the weight at the expense of good form and really feeling the shoulders perform the movement.
Hamstrings	Leg Curls or Good Mornings	3	5-3-1	Leg curls will work but if you're comfortable doing Good Mornings, these are an excellent posterior chain exercise that hit the hamstrings really well.
Calves	Standing or Seated Calf Raises	3	5-3-1	Use whichever exercise you didn't use on Day 2. Hold the top and bottom positions of the calf raise for at least 2 to 3 seconds to maximize the effect.
Traps	Barbell or Dumbbell Shrugs	3	5-3-1	Use a powerful, explosive movement for shrugs.
	Core Combo	4	-	2 sets of abs - 1 set of lower back - 1 set rotator cuff

General Comments:

- You'll be doing 3 sets for each body part...5 reps on the first set, 3 reps on the second set and 1 rep on the third set. Increase the weight on each set, unless you don't hit the target reps.
- Take 90 seconds to 2 minutes rest between each set.
- Don't push to failure on any sets. Always keep the do-or-die rep in you.

Your Written Notes:

_____

_____

_____

_____

Mad Scientist Muscle - Day 6 and 7 - Rest

Body part	Exercise	Sets	Reps	Notes
None				

Cardiovascular Training	
Activity	**Comment**
Aerobic Interval Training	This is an OPTIONAL cardio training session done on Day 6 <u>ONLY</u>. Go for 15 to 20 minutes using any of the work to rest intervals listed on the Aerobic Interval Training page, e.g. 2 minutes work to 30 seconds rest intervals. The idea here is not to push yourself hard but to just maintain cardio capacity.

General Comments:

- The cardio training for this day is optional. If you find that doing cardio slows down muscle growth, you can opt not to do it.

- From a nutritional standpoint, treat your cardio session as a regular training session and have a post-workout meal and supplementation.

Your Written Notes:

_____

_____

_____

Mad Scientist Muscle - Day 1 - Rest

Body part	Exercise	Sets	Reps	Notes
None				

General Comments:

Your Written Notes:

_____

_____

_____

Nick Nilsson

Mad Scientist Muscle - Day 2 - Rest

Body part	Exercise	Sets	Reps	Notes
None				

General Comments:

Your Written Notes:

_____

_____

_____

_____

Mad Scientist Muscle - Day 3 - Fun!

Body part	Exercise	Sets	Reps	Notes
Your choice!	Use whatever exercises you like today.			The only guideline here is to not push yourself to the maximum on any of your sets. You can absolutely train hard, but don't go to failure. We want to still be resting the nervous system in preparation for the Strength Testing on Day 5

General Comments:

- Today's training is all about fun...and it's optional, if you're really still trashed from the previous training.

- You choose from a variety of different exercises and techniques, as long as you don't push yourself to the maximum on any of your sets. This is the time to work on weak points and just try some new stuff.

- Take whatever rest periods you like...do whatever exercises you like...it's a free day to play in the gym.

- Aim for no more than 45 minutes of training on this day.

Your Written Notes:

_____

_____

_____

Mad Scientist Muscle - Day 4 - Rest

Body part	Exercise	Sets	Reps	Notes
None				

General Comments:

Your Written Notes:

_____

_____

_____

Mad Scientist Muscle - Day 5 - 1 Rep Max Testing

Exercise	Notes
Deadlifts	
Barbell Bench Press	
Squats or Front Squats	
Stiff-Legged Deadlifts	
Barbell Shoulder Press or Hang Clean and Press	
Barbell Curls	
Close Grip Bench Press	

General Comments:

- This day is all about maxing out. You're going to be doing very few sets here.

- When you're warming up for the max attempts, DO NOT do a whole bunch of sets or otherwise fatigue yourself. Your warm-up sets should be low-rep with lighter weight, gradually increasing but never pushing to the max until you're ready to really nail it. Your warm-ups should be "feelers" so you get a good idea of how much you're going to aim for on your max lift.

- We'll only be testing a few basic lifts here...the big three are here but you can choose whichever lifts you want to max out on to gauge your progress. **The above exercises are just suggestions.** You can also do these max attempts in any order you like. For example, if you really want to focus on what you can do on bench press, start with that. If deadlift is your focus, start with that.

- Pick 3 to 5 exercises from the list that you want to test. Don't try and do all of these!

Your Written Notes:

_____

_____

_____

_____

Mad Scientist Muscle - Day 6 and 7 - Rest

Body part	Exercise	Sets	Reps	Notes
None				

Cardiovascular Training	
Activity	**Comments**
Aerobic Interval Training	This is an OPTIONAL cardio training session done on Day 6 <u>ONLY.</u> Go for 15 to 20 minutes using any of the work to rest intervals listed on the Aerobic Interval Training page, e.g. 2 minutes work to 30 seconds rest intervals. The idea here is not to push yourself hard but to just maintain cardio capacity.

General Comments:

- The cardio training for this day is optional. If you find that doing cardio slows down muscle growth, you can opt not to do it.

- From a nutritional standpoint, treat your cardio session as a regular training session and have a post-workout meal and supplementation.

Your Written Notes:

_____

_____

_____

_____

Cycle 2 - Cluster Training

Week 1 - Structural

Week 2 - Volume - Cluster Training 1

Week 3 - Volume - Cluster Training 2

Week 4 - Volume - Cluster Training 3

Week 5 - Structural

Week 6 - Intensity - Single Rep Cluster Training 1

Week 7 - Intensity - Single Rep Cluster Training 2

Week 8 - OFF/Deload/Fun/Strength Test

Week 1
Structural Training

Day 1	Day 2	Day 3	Day 4	Day 5	Day 6 & 7
High-Rep Moderate Weight High-Speed Stretch sets	100's Stretch sets		Heavy Partial Training or High-Rep Partial Training	Heavy Partial Training or High- Rep Partial Training	
Back Chest Thighs Shoulders Hamstrings Biceps Triceps Calves	Chest Back Thighs Shoulders Hamstrings Biceps Triceps Calves	Rest	Chest Back Biceps Hamstrings	Triceps Shoulders Thighs Calves	Rest Cardio option

Nick Nilsson

Week 2 - Volume Cluster Training

During the three weeks of Cluster Training, we're going to be increasing the workload gradually as you go through the training sessions while at the same time, decreasing the amount of rest time in between sets. This is going to gradually move you towards overtraining, which is the goal of this phase.

The number in (), e.g. (1) is the number of Cluster sets you'll be doing for that body part. The numbers above are the number of mini-sets and reps you'll be doing, e.g. 5 x 3 means 5 mini-sets of 3 reps.

Day 1	Day 2	Day 3	Day 4	Day 5	Day 6 & 7
4 x 3 2 min rest	4 x 3 2 min rest		Pyramid Clusters 2 min rest	Pyramid Clusters 2 min rest	
Chest (2) Back (2) Biceps (1) Triceps (1)	Thighs (2) Shoulders (1) Hams (1) Calves (1) Traps (1)	Rest	Chest (2) Back (2) Biceps (1) Triceps (1)	Thighs (2) Shoulders (1) Hams (1) Calves (1) Traps (1)	Rest Cardio option

Week 3 -
Volume Cluster Training

Day 8	Day 9	Day 10	Day 11	Day 12	Day 13 & 14
5 x 3 90 sec rest	5 x 3 90 sec rest		Pyramid Clusters] 90 sec rest	Pyramid Clusters] 90 sec rest	
Chest (3) Back (3) Biceps (1) Triceps (1)	Thighs (3) Shoulders (1) Hams (1) Calves (1) Traps (1)	Rest	Chest (3) Back (3) Biceps (1) Triceps (1)	Thighs (3) Shoulders (1) Hams (1) Calves (1) Traps (1)	Rest Cardio option

Week 4 - Volume
Cluster Training

Day 15	Day 16	Day 17	Day 18	Day 19	Day 20 & 21
x 3 min rest	6 x 3 1 min rest		Pyramid Clusters] 1 min rest	Pyramid Clusters] 1 min rest	
est (3) ck (3) ceps (2) ceps (2)	Thighs (3) Shoulders (2) Hams (2) Calves (2)	Rest	Chest (3) Back (3) Biceps (2) Triceps (2)	Thighs (3) Shoulders (2) Hams (2) Calves (2))	Rest Cardio option

Week 5
Structural Training

Day 1	Day 2	Day 3	Day 4	Day 5	Day 6 & 7
igh-Rep oderate Weight igh-Speed tretch sets	100's Stretch sets		Heavy Partial Training or High-Rep Partial Training	Heavy Partial Training or High- Rep Partial Training	
ack hest highs houlders amstrings ceps iceps alves	Chest Back Thighs Shoulders Hamstrings Biceps Triceps Calves	Rest	Chest Back Biceps Hamstrings	Triceps Shoulders Thighs Calves	Rest Cardio option

Weeks 6 and 7 - IntensitySingle
Rep Cluster Training

We'll be doing the same set/rep scheme for both weeks of the Single Rep Cluster Training. When you've completed one week, you'll go through and repeat it the following week using the same exercises to achieve a training effect. Rep ranges are higher on the first two and lower on the second two days.

Day 1	Day 2	Day 3	Day 4	Day 5	Day 6 & 7
10-12 x 1 2 min rest	10-12 x 1 2 min rest		5-7 x 1 2 min rest Bottom-Start	5-7 x 1 2 min rest Bottom-Start	
Chest (2) Back (2) Biceps (1) Triceps (1)	Thighs (2) Shoulders (1) Hams (1) Calves (1) Traps (1)	Rest	Chest (2) Back (2) Biceps (1) Triceps (1)	Thighs (2) Shoulders (1) Hams (1) Calves (1)) Traps (1)	Rest Cardio option

Week 8 - OFF/Deload/Fun/Strength Test

Day 1	Day 2	Day 3	Day 4	Day 5	Day 6 & 7
Rest	Rest	Fun!	Rest	StrengthTest 1 RM's	Rest Cardio option

Mad Scientist Muscle - Day 1 - Cluster Training

Body part	Exercise	Rounds	Sets x Reps	Notes
Back	Bent-Over Barbell Rows, Seated Cable Rows or Deadlifts	2	4 x 3	When doing barbell rows, don't dip your upper body down to meet the bar. With cable rows, don't stretch forward by bending at the lower back - stretch forward by letting your shoulders pull forward. I prefer to save deadlifts for the Pyramid Cluster Training, but you can do them here instead, if you like.
Chest	Flat Barbell or Dumbbell Presses	2	4 x 3	Try to consciously squeeze your pecs as you press. Keep your feet planted firmly on the floor.
Biceps	Barbell Curls orDumbbell Curls	1	4 x 3	Use a controlled movement. The biceps won't grow if you swing the weight up without putting tension on them.
Triceps	Bar Dips, Lying Tricep Extensions or Close Grip Bench Press	1	4 x 3	Add weight to the bar dip if you need to. With extensions, keep your upper arms tilted slightly back to keep tension on the triceps throughout the movement.

General Comments:

- You will be using the Cluster Training training style today. This week, each Cluster set consists of 4 mini-sets of 3 reps with 10 seconds rest in between.

- Take 2 minutes rest in between each Cluster set.

- Stay strict with your 10 seconds in between mini-sets. If you need to, get someone to count it for you to keep you on track.

- Select a weight you can normally perform about 8 reps with for your Cluster Training for today.

Your Written Notes:

_____

_____

_____

Nick Nilsson

Mad Scientist Muscle - Day 2 - Cluster Training

Body part	Exercise	Rounds	Sets x Reps	Notes
Thighs/Quads	Squats, Lunges or Leg Press	2	4 x 3	Squats are preferable for Cluster Training on this day (if you didn't use deadlifts the day before). Lunges or Leg Press will also work, though.
Shoulders	Military Press or Seated Dumbbell Presses	1	4 x 3	When doing dumbbell presses, tilt the dumbbells down slightly as if if pouring water on your head. This keeps the tension on the delts far better.
Hamstrings	Stiff Legged Deadlifts or Leg Curlss	1	4 x 3	I prefer to set the weight back down on the floor between each rep, just like with regular deadlifts. It'll allow you to reset your lower back position on each rep and reduce back issues.
Calves	Standing or SeatedCalf Raises	1	4 x 3	Be sure to take the tension completely off the calves in between mini-sets by removing your feet from the machine. The 10 second rest is there to flush waste products out - if you still keep even a little tension on, the waste products won't get flushed.
Traps	Barbell or Dumbbell Shrugs	1	4 x 3	When doing shrugs, use an explosive movement out of the bottom. They're fast-twitch fibers that thrive on that.
	Core Combo	4	4 x 3	2 sets of abs - 1 set of lower back - 1 set rotator cuff

General Comments:

- You will be using the Cluster Training style today. This week, each Cluster set consists of 4 mini-sets of 3 reps with 10 seconds rest in between.

- Take 2 minutes rest in between each Cluster set.

- Stay strict with your 10 seconds in between mini-sets. If you need to, get someone to count it for you to keep you on track.

- Select a weight you can normally perform about 8 reps with for your Cluster Training for today.

- Select a weight you can normally perform about 8 reps with for your Cluster Training for today.

Your Written Notes:

_____

_____

Mad Scientist Muscle - Day 3 - Rest

Body part	Exercise	Sets	Reps	Notes
None				

Cardiovascular Training	
Activity	Comments

General Comments:

Your Written Notes:

_____

_____

_____

_____

Mad Scientist Muscle - Day 4 - Pyramid Cluster Training

Body part	Exercise	Rounds	Sets x Reps	Notes
Back	Deadlifts, Weighted Chins, or Pulldowns	2	1 x 1 1 x 2 1 x 3 1 x 2 1 x 1	Deadlifts are the preferred exercise for this day. They'll hit the most muscle mass.
Chest	Flat Barbell or Dumbbell Presses	1	1 x 1 1 x 2 1 x 3 1 x 2 1 x 1	Use whichever version of the bench press you DIDN'T use on the first day, e.g. if you did barbell presses on Day 1, then do dumbbell presses today.
Biceps	Barbell Curls orDumbbell Curls	1	1 x 1 1 x 2 1 x 3 1 x 2 1 x 1	Again, use whichever version of the curl you DIDN'T use on the first day.
Triceps	Bar Dips, Lying Tricep Extensions or Close Grip Bench Press	1	1 x 1 1 x 2 1 x 3 1 x 2 1 x 1	Add weight to the bar dip if you need to. With extensions, keep your upper arms tilted slightly back to keep tension on the triceps throughout the movement.

General Comments:

- You will be using the Pyramid Cluster Training training style today. This session, you will be ramping up and then down the reps on each set, 1 rep, 2 reps, 3 reps, 2 reps, 1 rep, with 10 seconds rest in between.

- Take 2 minutes rest in between each Cluster set.

- Stay strict with your 10 seconds in between mini-sets. If you need to, get someone to count it for you to keep you on track.

- Select a weight you can normally perform 5 reps with for your Cluster Training for today.

Your Written Notes:

_____

_____

_____

Mad Scientist Muscle - Day 5 - Pyramid Cluster Training

Body part	Exercise	Rounds	Sets x Reps	Notes
Thighs/ Quads	Front Squats, Split Squats, Leg Press, or Back Squats	2	1 x 1 1 x 2 1 x 3 1 x 2 1 x 1	If you used Squats on Day 2 and did Deadlifts on Day 4, go with a different leg exercise than back squats here. Front Squats are an excellent option - they're well-suited to this lower-rep training.
Shoulders	Hang Clean and Press, Military Press or Seated Dumbbell Presses	1	1 x 1 1 x 2 1 x 3 1 x 2 1 x 1	This is a good day to do Clean and Press, if you want some explosive work. They'll hit the traps strongly, too. Shoulders are worked after thighs here in case you decide to do Front Squats.
Hamstrings	Stiff Legged Deadlifts, Leg Curls or Good Mornings	1	1 x 1 1 x 2 1 x 3 1 x 2 1 x 1	To increase the stretch on the hams, set two 25-lb plates on the ground in front of the bar and put your forefeet area on them so you have a stretch in your calves. Only do Good Mornings if you're comfortable with the exercise.
Calves	Standing, Donkey or Seated Calf Raises	1	1 x 1 1 x 2 1 x 3 1 x 2 1 x 1	Take the tension off the calves in between mini-sets by removing your feet from the machine. The 10 second rest is there to flush waste products out. Use an exercise you didn't use last time.
Traps	Barbell or Dumbbell Shrugs	1	1 x 1 1 x 2 1 x 3 1 x 2 1 x 1	When doing shrugs, use an explosive movement out of the bottom. They're fast-twitch fibers that thrive on that.
	Core Combo	4	-	2 sets of abs - 1 set of lower back - 1 set rotator cuff

General Comments:

- You will be using the Pyramid Cluster Training training style today. This session, you will be ramping up and then down the reps on each set, 1 rep, 2 reps, 3 reps, 2 reps, 1 rep, with 10 seconds rest in between.

Nick Nilsson

- Take 2 minutes rest in between each Cluster set.

- Stay strict with your 10 seconds in between mini-sets. If you need to, get someone to count it for you to keep you on track.

- Select a weight you can normally perform 5 reps with for your Cluster Training for today.

Your Written Notes:

_____

_____

_____

Mad Scientist Muscle - Day 8 - Cluster Training

Body part	Exercise	Rounds	Sets x Reps	Notes
Back	Bent-Over Barbell Rows, Seated Cable Rows or Deadlifts	3	5 x 3	When doing barbell rows, don't dip your upper body down to meet the bar. With cable rows, don't stretch forward by bending at the lower back - stretch forward by letting your shoulders pull forward. I prefer to save deadlifts for the Pyramid Cluster Training, but you can do them here instead, if you like.
Chest	Flat Barbell or Dumbbell Presses	3	5 x 3	Try to consciously squeeze your pecs as you press. Keep your feet planted firmly on the floor.
Biceps	Barbell Curls orDumbbell Curls	1	5 x 3	Use a controlled movement. The biceps won't grow if you swing the weight up without putting tension on them.
Triceps	Bar Dips, Lying Tricep Extensions or Close Grip Bench Press	1	5 x 3	Add weight to the bar dip if you need to. With extensions, keep your upper arms tilted slightly back to keep tension on the triceps throughout the movement.

General Comments:

- You will be using the Cluster Training training style today. This week, each Cluster set consists of 5 mini-sets of 3 reps with 10 seconds rest in between.

- Take 90 seconds rest in between each Cluster set.

- Stay strict with your 10 seconds in between mini-sets. If you need to, get someone to count it for you to keep you on track.

- Select a weight you can normally perform about 8 reps with for your Cluster Training for today.

Your Written Notes:

___

___

Mad Scientist Muscle - Day 9 - Cluster Training

Body part	Exercise	Rounds	Sets x Reps	Notes
Thighs/ Quads	Squats, Lunges or Leg Press	3	5 x 3	Squats are preferable for Cluster Training on this day (if you didn't use deadlifts the day before). Lunges or Leg Press will also work, though.
Shoulders	Military Press or Seated Dumbbell Presses	1	5 x 3	When doing dumbbell presses, tilt the dumbbells down slightly as if if pouring water on your head. This keeps the tension on the delts far better.
Hamstrings	Stiff Legged Deadlifts or Leg Curls	1	5 x 3	I prefer to set the weight back down on the floor between each rep, just like with regular deadlifts. It'll allow you to reset your lower back position on each rep and reduce back issues.
Calves	Standing or SeatedCalf Raises	1	5 x 3	Be sure to take the tension completely off the calves in between mini-sets by removing your feet from the machine. The 10 second rest is there to flush waste products out - if you still keep even a little tension on, the waste products won't get flushed.
Traps	Barbell or Dumbbell Shrugs	1	5 x 3	When doing shrugs, use an explosive movement out of the bottom. They're fast-twitch fibers that thrive on that.
	Core Combo	4	-	2 sets of abs - 1 set of lower back - 1 set rotator cuff

General Comments:

- You will be using the Cluster Training style today. This week, each Cluster set consists of 5 mini-sets of 3 reps with 10 seconds rest in between.

- Take 90 seconds rest in between each Cluster set. Select a weight you can normally perform about 8 reps

- Stay strict with your 10 seconds in between mini-sets.

Your Written Notes:

_____

_____

Mad Scientist Muscle - Day 10 - Rest

Body part	Exercise	Sets	Reps	Notes
None				

Cardiovascular Training	
Activity	Comments

General Comments:

Your Written Notes:

_____

_____

_____

_____

Nick Nilsson

Mad Scientist Muscle - Day 11 - Pyramid Cluster Training

Body part	Exercise	Rounds	Sets x Reps	Notes
Back	Deadlifts, Weighted Chins, or Pulldowns	3	1 x 1 1 x 2 1 x 3 1 x 2 1 x 1	Deadlifts are the preferred exercise for this day. They'll hit the most muscle mass.
Chest	Flat Barbell or Dumbbell Presses	3	1 x 1 1 x 2 1 x 3 1 x 2 1 x 1	Use whichever version of the bench press you DIDN'T use on the first day, e.g. if you did barbell presses on Day 1, then do dumbbell presses today.
Biceps	Barbell Curls orDumbbell Curls	1	1 x 1 1 x 2 1 x 3 1 x 2 1 x 1	Again, use whichever version of the curl you DIDN'T use on the first day.
Triceps	Bar Dips, Lying Tricep Extensions or Close Grip Bench Press	1	1 x 1 1 x 2 1 x 3 1 x 2 1 x 1	Add weight to the bar dip if you need to. With extensions, keep your upper arms tilted slightly back to keep tension on the triceps throughout the movement.

General Comments:

- You will be using the Pyramid Cluster Training training style today. This session, you will be ramping up and then down the reps on each set, 1 rep, 2 reps, 3 reps, 2 reps, 1 rep, with 10 seconds rest in between.

- Take 90 seconds rest in between each Cluster set.

- Stay strict with your 10 seconds in between mini-sets. If you need to, get someone to count it for you to keep you on track.

- Select a weight you can normally perform 5 reps with for your Cluster Training for today.

Your Written Notes:

_____

_____

Mad Scientist Muscle - Day 12 - Pyramid Cluster Training

Body part	Exercise	Rounds	Sets x Reps	Notes
Thighs/ Quads	Front Squats, Split Squats, Leg Press, or Back Squats	3	1 x 1 1 x 2 1 x 3 1 x 2 1 x 1	Deadlifts are the preferred exercise for this day. They'll hit the most muscle mass.
Shoulders	Hang Clean and Press, Military Press or Seated Dumbbell Presses	1	1 x 1 1 x 2 1 x 3 1 x 2 1 x 1	Use whichever version of the bench press you DIDN'T use on the first day, e.g. if you did barbell presses on Day 1, then do dumbbell presses today.
Hamstrings	Stiff Legged Deadlifts, Leg Curls or Good Mornings	1	1 x 1 1 x 2 1 x 3 1 x 2 1 x 1	Again, use whichever version of the curl you DIDN'T use on the first day.
Calves	Standing, Donkey or SeatedCalf Raises	1	1 x 1 1 x 2 1 x 3 1 x 2 1 x 1	Add weight to the bar dip if you need to. With extensions, keep your upper arms tilted slightly back to keep tension on the triceps throughout the movement.
Traps	Barbell or Dumbbell Shrugs	1	1 x 1 1 x 2 1 x 3 1 x 2 1 x 1	When doing shrugs, use an explosive movement out of the bottom. They're fast-twitch fibers that thrive on that.
	Core Combo	4	-	2 sets of abs - 1 set of lower back - 1 set rotator cuff

General Comments:

- You will be using the Pyramid Cluster Training training style today. This session, you will be ramping up and then down the reps on each set, 1 rep, 2 reps, 3 reps, 2 reps, 1 rep, with 10 seconds rest in between.

- Take 90 seconds rest in between each Cluster set.

- Stay strict with your 10 seconds in between mini-sets. If you need to, get someone to count it for you to keep you on track.

- Select a weight you can normally perform 5 reps with for your Cluster Training for today.

Your Written Notes:

_____

_____

Nick Nilsson

Mad Scientist Muscle - Day 13 & 14 - Rest

Body part	Exercise	Sets	Reps	Notes
None				

Cardiovascular Training	
Activity	**Comments**
Aerobic Interval Training	This is an OPTIONAL cardio training session done on Day 13 <u>ONLY</u>. Go for 15 to 20 minutes using any of the work to rest intervals listed on the Aerobic Interval Training page, e.g. 2 minutes work to 30 seconds rest intervals. The idea here is not to push yourself hard but to just maintain cardio capacity.

General Comments:

- The cardio training for this day is optional. If you find that doing cardio slows down muscle growth, you can opt not to do it.

- From a nutritional standpoint, treat your cardio session as a regular training session and have a post-workout meal and supplementation.

Your Written Notes:

_____

_____

_____

_____

Mad Scientist Muscle - Day 15 - Cluster Training

Body part	Exercise	Rounds	Sets x Reps	Notes
Back	Bent-Over Barbell Rows, Seated Cable Rows or Deadlifts	3	6 x 3	When doing barbell rows, don't dip your upper body down to meet the bar. With cable rows, don't stretch forward by bending at the lower back - stretch forward by letting your shoulders pull forward. I prefer to save deadlifts for the Pyramid Cluster Training, but you can do them here instead, if you like.
Chest	Flat Barbell or Dumbbell Presses	3	6 x 3	Try to consciously squeeze your pecs as you press. Keep your feet planted firmly on the floor.
Biceps	Barbell Curls orDumbbell Curls	2	6 x 3	Use a controlled movement. The biceps won't grow if you swing the weight up without putting tension on them.
Triceps	Bar Dips, Lying Tricep Extensions or Close Grip Bench Press	2	6 x 3	Add weight to the bar dip if you need to. With extensions, keep your upper arms tilted slightly back to keep tension on the triceps throughout the movement.

General Comments:

- You will be using the Cluster Training training style today. This week, each Cluster set consists of 6 mini-sets of 3 reps with 10 seconds rest in between.

- Take 1 minute rest in between each Cluster set.

- Stay strict with your 10 seconds in between mini-sets. If you need to, get someone to count it for you to keep you on track.

- Select a weight you can normally perform about 9-10 reps with for your Cluster Training for today.

Your Written Notes:

_____

_____

_____

Nick Nilsson

Mad Scientist Muscle - Day 16 - Cluster Training

Body part	Exercise	Rounds	Sets x Reps	Notes
Thighs/ Quads	Squats, Lunges or Leg Press	3	6 x 3	Squats are preferable for Cluster Training on this day (if you didn't use deadlifts the day before). Lunges or Leg Press will also work, though.
Shoulders	Military Press or Seated Dumbbell Presses	2	6 x 3	When doing dumbbell presses, tilt the dumbbells down slightly as if if pouring water on your head. This keeps the tension on the delts far better.
Hamstrings	Stiff Legged Deadlifts or Leg Curls	2	6 x 3	I prefer to set the weight back down on the floor between each rep, just like with regular deadlifts. It'll allow you to reset your lower back position on each rep and reduce back issues.
Calves	Standing or SeatedCalf Raises	2	6 x 3	Be sure to take the tension completely off the calves in between mini-sets by removing your feet from the machine. The 10 second rest is there to flush waste products out - if you still keep even a little tension on, the waste products won't get flushed.
	Core Combo	4	-	2 sets of abs - 1 set of lower back - 1 set rotator cuff

General Comments:

- You will be using the Cluster Training style today. This week, each Cluster set consists of 6 mini-sets of 3 reps with 10 seconds rest in between. Take 90 seconds rest in between each Cluster set.

- Take 1 minute rest in between each Cluster set.

- Stay strict with your 10 seconds in between mini-sets. If you need to, get someone to count it for you to keep you on track.

- Select a weight you can normally perform about 9-10 reps with for your Cluster Training for today.

Your Written Notes:

_____

_____

_____

Mad Scientist Muscle - Day 17 - Rest

Body part	Exercise	Sets	Reps	Notes
None				

Cardiovascular Training	
Activity	Comments

General Comments:

Your Written Notes:

_____

_____

_____

_____

Nick Nilsson

Mad Scientist Muscle - Day 18 - Pyramid Cluster Training

Body part	Exercise	Rounds	Sets x Reps	Notes
Back	Deadlifts, Weighted Chins, or Pulldowns	3	1 x 1 1 x 2 1 x 3 1 x 2 1 x 1	When doing barbell rows, don't dip your upper body down to meet the bar. With cable rows, don't stretch forward by bending at the lower back - stretch forward by letting your shoulders pull forward. I prefer to save deadlifts for the Pyramid Cluster Training, but you can do them here instead, if you like.
Chest	Flat Barbell or Dumbbell Presses	3	1 x 1 1 x 2 1 x 3 1 x 2 1 x 1	Try to consciously squeeze your pecs as you press. Keep your feet planted firmly on the floor.
Biceps	Barbell Curls orDumbbell Curls	2	1 x 1 1 x 2 1 x 3 1 x 2 1 x 1	Use a controlled movement. The biceps won't grow if you swing the weight up without putting tension on them.
Triceps	Bar Dips, Lying Tricep Extensions or Close Grip Bench Press	2	1 x 1 1 x 2 1 x 3 1 x 2 1 x 1	Add weight to the bar dip if you need to. With extensions, keep your upper arms tilted slightly back to keep tension on the triceps throughout the movement.

General Comments:

- You will be using the Pyramid Cluster Training training style today. This session, you will be ramping up and then down the reps on each set, 1 rep, 2 reps, 3 reps, 2 reps, 1 rep, with 10 seconds rest in between.

- Take 1 minute rest in between each Cluster set.

- Stay strict with your 10 seconds in between mini-sets. If you need to, get someone to count it for you to keep you on track.

- Select a weight you can normally perform 5-6 reps with for your Cluster Training for today.

Your Written Notes:

_____

_____

_____

Mad Scientist Muscle - Day 19 - Pyramid Cluster Training

Body part	Exercise	Rounds	Sets x Reps	Notes
Thighs/ Quads	Front Squats, Split Squats, Leg Press, or Back Squats	3	1 x 1 1 x 2 1 x 3 1 x 2 1 x 1	If you used Squats on Day 2 and did Deadlifts on Day 4, go with a different leg exercise than back squats here. Front Squats are an excellent option - they're well-suited to this lower-rep training.
Shoulders	Hang Clean and Press, Military Press or Seated Dumbbell Presses	2	1 x 1 1 x 2 1 x 3 1 x 2 1 x 1	This is a good day to do Clean and Press, if you want some explosive work. They'll hit the traps strongly, too. Shoulders are worked after thighs here in case you decide to do Front Squats.
Hamstrings	Stiff Legged Deadlifts, Leg Curls or Good Mornings	2	1 x 1 1 x 2 1 x 3 1 x 2 1 x 1	To increase the stretch on the hams, set two 25-lb plates on the ground in front of the bar and put your forefeet area on them so you have a stretch in your calves. Only do Good Mornings if you're comfortable with the exercise.
Calves	Standing, Donkey or SeatedCalf Raises	2	1 x 1 1 x 2 1 x 3 1 x 2 1 x 1	Be sure to take the tension completely off the calves in between mini-sets by removing your feet from the machine. The 10 second rest is there to flush waste products out - if you still keep even a little tension on, the waste products won't get flushed. Use an exercise you didn't use last time.
	Core Combo	4	-	2 sets of abs - 1 set of lower back - 1 set rotator cuff

General Comments:

- You will be using the Pyramid Cluster Training training style today. This session, you will be ramping up and then down the reps on each set, 1 rep, 2 reps, 3 reps, 2 reps, 1 rep, with 10 seconds rest in between.

- Take 1 minute rest in between each Cluster set. Select a weight you can normally perform 5-6 reps

- Stay strict with your 10 seconds in between mini-sets.

Your Written Notes:

_____

_____

_____

Nick Nilsson

Mad Scientist Muscle - Day 20 & 21 - Rest

Body part	Exercise	Sets	Reps	Notes
None				

Cardiovascular Training	
Activity	**Comments**
Aerobic Interval Training	This is an OPTIONAL cardio training session done on Day 20 <u>ONLY</u>. Go for 15 to 20 minutes using any of the work to rest intervals listed on the Aerobic Interval Training page, e.g. 2 minutes work to 30 seconds rest intervals. The idea here is not to push yourself hard but to just maintain cardio capacity.

General Comments:

- The cardio training for this day is optional. If you find that doing cardio slows down muscle growth, you can opt not to do it.

- From a nutritional standpoint, treat your cardio session as a regular training session and have a post-workout meal and supplementation.

Your Written Notes:

_____

_____

_____

_____

Mad Scientist Muscle - Day 1 - Single Rep Cluster Training

Body part	Exercise	Rounds	Sets/ Reps	Notes
Chest	Flat Barbell Bench Press or Dumbbell Press	2	(10-12) x 1	Barbells are much better for performing this style of training. You can re-rack on every rep rather than having to get dumbbells into position on every single rep. Only use dumbbells for this style of training if you either have no choice or you have Power Hooks that allow you to hang the dumbbells from a bar.
Back	Deadlifts, Barbell Rows or Weighted Chin-Ups	2	(10-12) x 1	When using heavier weights on deadlifts, pull the bend into the bar first, before trying to lift it off the ground. If you pop it off, the plates will bounce back down. You can also choose to save deadlifts for the lower-rep day, if you wish.
Biceps	Barbell Curls	1	(10-12) x 1	Keep your knees bent and don't hunch forward.
Triceps	Close Grip Bench Press (flat or decline) or Weighted Dips	1	(10-12) x 1	When doing close grip, set your hands about shoulder width apart and keep your elbows tucked in to your sides.
	Core Combo	4	-	2 sets of abs - 1 set of lower back - 1 set rotator cuff

General Comments:

- You will be using the Single Rep Cluster Training training style today. This week, each Cluster set consists of 10-12 mini-sets of 1 rep with 10 seconds rest in between. I've given a range to shoot for rather than a specific number so that if you hit 10 but have a few more left in you, you can keep going. Keep the do-or-die reps in you, though.

- Take 2 minutes rest in between each Cluster set.

- Stay strict with your 10 seconds in between mini-sets. If you need to, get someone to count it for you to keep you on track.

- Select a weight you can normally perform about 5-7 "straight-through" reps with for your Cluster Training for today.

Your Written Notes:

_____

_____

Nick Nilsson

Mad Scientist Muscle - Day 2 - Single Rep Cluster Training

Body part	Exercise	Rounds	Sets/ Reps	Notes
Thighs	Front Squats, Split Squats or Leg Press	2	(10-12) x 1	Front squats will build up your core in addition to hitting the quads hard.
Shoulders	Military Press or DB Press	2	(10-12) x 1	The barbell military press will be a better option than dumbbells as you can just rerack the weight on each rep. Use dumbbells if the barbell press is not a good option.
Hamstrings	Stiff-Legged Deadlifts	1	(10-12) x 1	To focus even more on the hamstrings, set your forefoot area
Calves	Standing or Seated Calf Raises	1	(10-12) x 1	Hold the top and bottom positions of the calf raise for at least 2 to 3 seconds to maximize the effect.
Traps	Barbell or Dumbbell Shrugs	1	(10-12) x 1	Use a powerful, explosive movement for shrugs.
	Core Combo	4	-	2 sets of abs - 1 set of lower back - 1 set rotator cuff

General Comments:

- You will be using the Single Rep Cluster Training training style today. This week, each Cluster set consists of 10-12 mini-sets of 1 rep with 10 seconds rest in between. I've given a range to shoot for rather than a specific number so that if you hit 10 but have a few more left in you, you can keep going. Keep the do-or-die reps in you, though.

- Take 2 minutes rest in between each Cluster set.

- Stay strict with your 10 seconds in between mini-sets. If you need to, get someone to count it for you to keep you on track.

- Select a weight you can normally perform about 5-7 "straight-through" reps with for your Cluster Training for today.

Your Written Notes:

_____

_____

_____

Mad Scientist Muscle - Day 3 - Rest

Body part	Exercise	Sets	Reps	Notes
None				

Cardiovascular Training	
Activity	Comments

General Comments:

Your Written Notes:

Mad Scientist Muscle - Day 4 - Bottom-Start Single Rep Cluster Training

Body part	Exercise	Rounds	Sets/ Reps	Notes
Chest	Incline or Decline Barbell Bench Press or Dumbbell Press	2	(5-7) x 1	Use the version you didn't use on the first day. Barbells will be a better choice so you don't have to pick up the dumbbells every rep. Using barbells is the only real way to do bottom-start training as well.
Back	Weighted Chin-Ups, One Arm Dumbbell Rows, Barbell Rows or Deadlifts	2	(5-7) x 1	If you did deadlifts on the first day and will be doing squats the next day, use a row or other pulling movement rather than deadlifts. The Barbell Row is good to use the Bottom-Start technique with. Deadlifts are always bottom-start, so that'll be perfect, if that's your exercise.
Biceps	Dumbbell Curls or Preacher Curls	1	(5-7) x 1	When doing dumbbell curls, go one arm at a time in an alternating fashion, not both. You'll be able to lift more and with better form. Preacher Curls work well with the Bottom-Start technique.
Triceps	Close Grip Bench Press (flat or decline), Lying Tricep Extensions or Weighted Dips	1	(5-7) x 1	Use the exercise you didn't use on Day 1 for triceps. Decline close grip bench press works extremely well for loading the triceps. You can use the extensions for bottom-start training. Weighted dips can be done by standing on the floor at the bottom.
	Core Combo	4	-	2 sets of abs - 1 set of lower back - 1 set rotator cuff

General Comments:

- If you can, you will be using the Bottom-Start Single Rep Cluster Training training style today, otherwise just follow the normal single-rep style. Each Cluster set consists of 5-7 mini-sets of 1 rep with 10 seconds rest in between. I've given a range to shoot for rather than a specific number so that if you hit 5 but have a few more left in you, you can keep going. Keep the do-or-die reps in you.

- Where possible, start each rep from the BOTTOM of the movement, removing the elastic tension from the muscles, forcing them to take 100% of the load.

- Take 2 minutes rest in between each Cluster set.

- Stay strict with your 10 seconds in between mini-sets.

- Select a weight you can normally perform about 3-4 "straight-through" reps with.

Your Written Notes:

_____

_____

Mad Scientist Muscle - Day 5 - Single Rep Cluster Training

Body part	Exercise	Rounds	Sets/Reps	Notes
Thighs	Barbell Squats, Front Squats, DB Split Squats or Leg Press	2	(5-7) x 1	Barbell Back Squats or Front Squats are the best choice here. Both can be done very effectively with the bottom-start technique. Use the DB exercise or leg press if you can't do either of those here.
Shoulders	Hang Clean & Press, Military Press, or Seated DB Shoulder Presses	1	(5-7) x 1	Military Press (seated or standing) works great with bottom-start training. The Hang Clean and Press works great for low-rep power training like this.
Hamstrings	Stiff-Legged Deadlifts, Good Mornings or Leg Curls	1	(5-7) x 1	Use SLDLs as bottom-start training off the floor. Leg curls will work but if you're ok doing Good Mornings, these are a good posterior chain exercise that hit the hamstrings.
Calves	Standing or Seated Calf Raises	1	(5-7) x 1	Use whichever exercise you didn't use on Day 2. Hold the top and bottom positions of the calf raise for at least 2 to 3 seconds to maximize the effect. Start each rep from a big stretch.
Traps	Barbell or Dumbbell Shrugs	1	(5-7) x 1	Use a powerful, explosive movement for shrugs.
	Core Combo	4	-	2 sets of abs - 1 set of lower back - 1 set rotator cuff

General Comments:

- If you can, you will be using the Bottom-Start Single Rep Cluster Training training style today, otherwise just follow the normal single-rep style. Each Cluster set consists of 5-7 mini-sets of 1 rep with 10 seconds rest in between. I've given a range to shoot for rather than a specific number so that if you hit 5 but have a few more left in you, you can keep going. Keep the do-or-die reps in you.

- Where appropriate, you will start each rep from the BOTTOM of the movement, removing the elastic tension from the muscles, forcing them to take 100% of the load.

- Take 2 minutes rest in between each Cluster set.

- Stay strict with your 10 seconds in between mini-sets.

- Select a weight you can normally perform about 3-4 "straight-through" reps with.

Your Written Notes:

_____

_____

Mad Scientist Muscle - Day 6 and 7 - Rest

Body part	Exercise	Sets	Reps	Notes
None				

Cardiovascular Training	
Activity	**Comments**
Aerobic Interval Training	This is an OPTIONAL cardio training session done on Day 6 <u>ONLY</u>. Go for 15 to 20 minutes using any of the work to rest intervals listed on the Aerobic Interval Training page, e.g. 2 minutes work to 30 seconds rest intervals. The idea here is not to push yourself hard but to just maintain cardio capacity.

General Comments:

- The cardio training for this day is optional. If you find that doing cardio slows down muscle growth, you can opt not to do it.

- From a nutritional standpoint, treat your cardio session as a regular training session and have a post-workout meal and supplementation.

Your Written Notes:

_____

_____

_____

_____

Cycle 3 - Rest-Pause Training

Week 1 - Structural

Week 2 - Volume - Rest-Pause Training 1

Week 3 - Volume - Rest-Pause Training 2

Week 4 - Volume - Rest-Pause Training 3

Week 5 - Structural

Week 6 - Intensity - Triple Add Sets 1

Week 7 - Intensity - Triple Add Sets 2

Week 8 - OFF/Deload/Fun/Strength Test

Week 1
Structural Training

Day 1	Day 2	Day 3	Day 4	Day 5	Day 6 & 7
High-Rep Moderate Weight High-Speed Stretch sets	100's Stretch sets		Heavy Partial Training or High-Rep Partial Training	Heavy Partial Training or High- Rep Partial Training	
Back Chest Thighs Shoulders Hamstrings Biceps Triceps Calves	Chest Back Thighs Shoulders Hamstrings Biceps Triceps Calves	Rest	Chest Back Biceps Hamstrings	Triceps Shoulders Thighs Calves	Rest Cardio option

Nick Nilsson

Week 2 - Volume Rest-Pause Training

With Rest-Pause Training, the "10 rep start" means the first set will be for 10 reps, then you'll continue with rest-pause from there. When it says "5 rep start" that means your first set will be 5 reps then continue with rest-pause from there. We'll be increasing the number of rest-pause sets done, while decreasing rest periods between sets.

Day 1	Day 2	Day 3	Day 4	Day 5	Day 6 & 7
10 rep start 2 min rest	10 rep start 2 min rest		5 rep start 2 min rest	5 rep start 2 min rest	
Back (2) Chest (2) Biceps (1) Calves (1)	Triceps (1) Thighs (2) Shoulders (1) Hams (1) Traps (1)	Rest	Chest (2) Back (2) Biceps (1) Calves (1)	Shoulders (1) Triceps (1) Thighs (2) Hams (1) Traps (1)	Rest Cardio option

Week 3 - VolumeRest-Pause Training

I recommend using the same exercises you used the previous week so you can better gauge your progress and get a good training effect on the muscles. By sticking with the same exercises, your muscles will have an easier time adapting and you'll also have a good idea of what weights to use.

Day 8	Day 9	Day 10	Day 11	Day 12	Day 13 & 14
10 rep start 90 sec rest	10 rep start 90 sec rest		5 rep start 90 sec rest	5 rep start 90 sec rest	
Back (3) Chest (3) Biceps (1) Calves (1)	Triceps (1) Thighs (3) Shoulders (1) Hams (1) Traps (1)	Rest	Chest (3) Back (3) Biceps (1) Calves (1)	Shoulders (1) Triceps (1) Thighs (3) Hams (1) Traps (1)	Rest Cardio option

Week 4 - Volume Rest-Pause Training

On this final week, you'll be maximizing the training volume while minimizing rest periods. Continue with the same exercises you used on the previous weeks. You should make an effort to try and increase your weights whenever possible, even though the rest is decreasing.

Day 15	Day 16	Day 17	Day 18	Day 19	Day 20 & 21
10 rep start 1 min rest	10 rep start 1 min rest		5 rep start 1 min rest	5 rep start 1 min rest	
Back (3) Chest (3) Biceps (2) Calves (2)	Triceps (2) Thighs (3) Shoulders (2) Hams (2) Traps (1)	Rest	Chest (3) Back (3) Biceps (2) Calves (2)	Shoulders (2) Triceps (2) Thighs (3) Hams (2) Traps (1)	Rest Cardio option

Week 5 Structural Training

Day 1	Day 2	Day 3	Day 4	Day 5	Day 6 & 7
High-Rep Moderate Weight High-Speed Stretch sets	100's Stretch sets		Heavy Partial Training or High-Rep Partial Training	Heavy Partial Training or High- Rep Partial Training	
Back Chest Thighs Shoulders Hamstrings Biceps Triceps Calves	Chest Back Thighs Shoulders Hamstrings Biceps Triceps Calves	Rest	Chest Back Biceps Hamstrings	Triceps Shoulders Thighs Calves	Rest Cardio option

Nick Nilsson

Weeks 6 and 7 - Intensity
Triple Add Sets and Low Rep Strength Training

We'll be doing the same set/rep scheme for both weeks of the Triple Add Set Training. The first two days will be done using Triple Add Sets. The second two training days will be Low Rep Strength Training. Triple Add Sets are a powerful technique and repeating it twice in a week will actually push you back towards overtraining, which is why you'll be doing Low-Rep Strength Training for the second two days instead.

Day 1	Day 2	Day 3	Day 4	Day 5	Day 6 & 7
Triple Add Sets 2 min rest	Triple Add Sets 2 min rest		Low-Rep Strength 2 min rest	Low-Rep Strength 2 min rest	
Chest (2) Back (2) Biceps (2) Triceps (2)	Thighs (2) Shoulders (2) Hams (2) Calves (1) Traps (1)	Rest	Chest Back Biceps Triceps	Thighs Shoulders Hamstrings Calves Traps	Rest Cardio option

Week 8 - OFF/Deload/Fun/Strength Test

Day 1	Day 2	Day 3	Day 4	Day 5	Day 6 & 7
Rest	Rest	Rest	Rest	StrengthTest 1 RM's	Rest Cardio option

Mad Scientist Muscle - Day 1 - Rest-Pause Training

Body part	Exercise	Rounds	Reps	Notes
Back	Deadlifts, Chin-Ups, Barbell Rows or One-Arm Dumbbell Rows	2	10-x-x	Deadlifts are the preferred exercise here since they involve the most muscle mass.
Chest	Barbell Bench Press or Dumbbell Bench Press	2	10-x-x	When doing barbell bench, be sure you don't flare your elbows out wide to the side at the bottom. Keep them tucked in towards your body a bit to save your shoulders.
Biceps	Barbell, Preacher or Dumbbell Curls	1	10-x-x	Any of these exercises is fine here. You're just doing one rest-pause set so make it count.
Calves	Standing, Donkey or Seated Calf Raises	1	10-x-x	When doing calf raises, hold the stretch at the bottom and the contraction at the top for a few seconds each, to maxmize the tension on the calves.
	Core Combo	4	-	2 sets of abs - 1 set of lower back - 1 set rotator cuff

General Comments:

- You will be using the Rest-Pause Training style today. Start with 10 reps on your first set, then rest 20 seconds, then go back to the same exercise and get as many more reps as you can (this might be about 3 to 5 reps - this is the "x" in the Reps section), rest 20 seconds, then get as many more reps as you can (maybe 2 to 3 reps).

- One time through these three sections is ONE rest-pause set.

- Take 2 minutes rest between rest-pause sets here.

Your Written Notes:

_____

_____

_____

_____

Nick Nilsson

Mad Scientist Muscle - Day 2 - Rest-Pause Training

Body part	Exercise	Rounds	Reps	Notes
Triceps	Weighted Dips, Close Grip Bench Press or Lying Tricep Extensions	1	10-x-x	Dips are the preferred exercise here. Keep your elbows in close to your body and keep your torso upright in order to focus the stress on the triceps over the chest.
Thighs	Front Squats or Dumbbell Split Squats	2	10-x-x	The preferred exercise here is the Front Squat. If you use DB Split Squats, do 10 reps on one leg, then 10 reps on the other, then take 20 sec, then go again. Switch legs that you start with on the next set to keep things even.
Shoulders	Dumbbell Shoulder Press	1	10-x-x	A good technique is to sit backwards in the Preacher bench so that the pad hits you in the mid-back rather than using the shoulder press bench with the vertical back. You'll get more back support this way.
Hamstrings	Leg Curls or Stiff-Legged Deadlifts	1	10-x-x	Leg Curls are a good option here as we can save the Stiff-Legged Deadlifts for the lower-rep day, which they're more suited to.
Traps	Barbell or Dumbbell Shrugs	1	10-x-x	With barbell shrugs, grip assistance is a good idea so that you work the traps without grip becoming an issue.
	Core Combo	4	-	2 sets of abs - 1 set of lower back - 1 set rotator cuff

General Comments:

- You will be using the Rest-Pause Training style today. Start with 10 reps on your first set, then rest 20 seconds, then go back to the same exercise and get as many more reps as you can (this might be about 3 to 5 reps - this is the "x" in the Reps section), rest 20 seconds, then get as many more reps as you can (maybe 2 to 3 reps).

- One time through these three sections is ONE rest-pause set.

- Take 2 minutes rest between rest-pause sets here

Your Written Notes:

_____

_____

Mad Scientist Muscle - Day 3 - Rest

Body part	Exercise	Sets	Reps	Notes
None				

Cardiovascular Training	
Activity	Comments

General Comments:

Your Written Notes:

_____

_____

_____

_____

Nick Nilsson

Mad Scientist Muscle - Day 4 - Rest-Pause Training

Body part	Exercise	Rounds	Reps	Notes
Chest	Incline/Decline Barbell Bench Press or Dumbbell Bench Press	2	5-x-x	Dumbbell bench press can be done on the Swiss ball here. If you decide to go with barbell presses, use either Incline or Decline, to switch it up from the flat bench.
Back	Weighted Chin-Ups, Pulldowns, Barbell Rows, One-Arm Dumbbell Rows or Deadlifts	2	5-x-x	If you did Deadlifts on Day 1, go with one of the other exercises here, and go with Squats tomorrow.
Biceps	Barbell, Preacher or Dumbbell Curls	1	5-x-x	Any of these exercises is fine here. You're just doing one rest-pause set so make it count.
Calves	Standing, Donkey or Seated Calf Raises	1	5-x-x	When doing calf raises, hold the stretch at the bottom and the contraction at the top for a few seconds each, to maxmize the tension on the calves.
	Core Combo	4	-	2 sets of abs - 1 set of lower back - 1 set rotator cuff

General Comments:

- You will be using the Rest-Pause Training style today. Start with 5 reps on your first set, then rest 20 seconds, then go back to the same exercise and get as many more reps as you can (this might be about 2-3 reps - this is the "x" in the Reps section), rest 20 seconds, then get as many more reps as you can (maybe 1 or 2 reps).

- One time through these three sections is ONE rest-pause set.

- Take 2 minutes rest between rest-pause sets here.

Your Written Notes:

_____

_____

_____

_____

Mad Scientist Muscle - Day 5 - Rest-Pause Training

Body part	Exercise	Rounds	Reps	Notes
Shoulders	Barbell Hang Clean and Press or Military Press	1	5-x-x	The Hang Clean and Press is a good one here. It's better suited to lower-rep, explosive training.
Triceps	Decline Close Grip Bench Press or Weighted Dips	1	5-x-x	Decline Close Grip Press is great for loading the triceps with heavy weight. You can also use flat Close Grip Press, if you prefer.
Thighs	Squats or Leg Press	2	5-x-x	The preferred exercise here is the Squat. Leg Press will work if you're not physically able to squat, but you'll get more out of the Barbell Squat as an overall mass-builder.
Hamstrings	Stiff-Legged Deadlifts or Leg Curls	1	5-x-x	Stiff-Legged Deadlifts are the preferred option here. They're well-suited to lower-rep, heavier training.
Traps	Barbell or Dumbbell Shrugs	1	5-x-x	With barbell shrugs, grip assistance is a good idea so that you work the traps without grip becoming an issue.
	Core Combo	4	-	2 sets of abs - 1 set of lower back - 1 set rotator cuff

General Comments:

- You will be using the Rest-Pause Training style today. Start with 5 reps on your first set, then rest 20 seconds, then go back to the same exercise and get as many more reps as you can (this might be about 2-3 reps - this is the "x" in the Reps section), rest 20 seconds, then get as many more reps as you can (maybe 1 or 2 reps).

- One time through these three sections is ONE rest-pause set.

- Take 2 minutes rest between rest-pause sets here.

Your Written Notes:

_____

_____

_____

_____

Mad Scientist Muscle - Day 6 & 7 - Rest

Body part	Exercise	Sets	Reps	Notes
None				

Cardiovascular Training	
Activity	**Comments**
Aerobic Interval Training	This is an OPTIONAL cardio training session done on Day 6 <u>ONLY</u>. Go for 15 to 20 minutes using any of the work to rest intervals listed on the Aerobic Interval Training page, e.g. 2 minutes work to 30 seconds rest intervals. The idea here is not to push yourself hard but to just maintain cardio capacity.

General Comments:

- The cardio training for this day is optional. If you find that doing cardio slows down muscle growth, you can opt not to do it.

- From a nutritional standpoint, treat your cardio session as a regular training session and have a post-workout meal and supplementation.

Your Written Notes:

_____

_____

_____

_____

Mad Scientist Muscle - Day 8 - Rest-Pause Training

Body part	Exercise	Rounds	Reps	Notes
Back	Deadlifts, Chin-Ups, Barbell Rows or One-Arm Dumbbell Rows	3	10-x-x	Deadlifts are the preferred exercise here since they involve the most muscle mass.
Chest	Barbell Bench Press or Dumbbell Bench Press	3	10-x-x	When doing barbell bench, be sure you don't flare your elbows out wide to the side at the bottom. Keep them tucked in towards your body a bit to save your shoulders.
Biceps	Barbell, Preacher or Dumbbell Curls	1	10-x-x	Any of these exercises is fine here. You're just doing one rest-pause set so make it count.
Calves	Standing, Donkey or Seated Calf Raises	1	10-x-x	When doing calf raises, hold the stretch at the bottom and the contraction at the top for a few seconds each, to maxmize the tension on the calves.
	Core Combo	4	-	2 sets of abs - 1 set of lower back - 1 set rotator cuff

General Comments:

- You will be using the Rest-Pause Training style today. Start with 10 reps on your first set, then rest 20 seconds, then go back to the same exercise and get as many more reps as you can (this might be about 3 to 5 reps - this is the "x" in the Reps section), rest 20 seconds, then get as many more reps as you can (maybe 2 to 3 reps).

- One time through these three sections is ONE rest-pause set.

- Take 90 seconds rest between rest-pause sets here.

Your Written Notes:

_____

_____

_____

_____

Nick Nilsson

Mad Scientist Muscle - Day 9 - Rest-Pause Training

Body part	Exercise	Rounds	Reps	Notes
Triceps	Weighted Dips, Close Grip Bench Press or Lying Tricep Extensions	1	10-x-x	Dips are the preferred exercise here. Keep your elbows in close to your body and keep your torso upright in order to focus the stress on the triceps over the chest.
Thighs	Front Squats or Dumbbell Split Squats	3	10-x-x	The preferred exercise here is the Front Squat. If you use DB Split Squats, do 10 reps on one leg, then 10 reps on the other, then take 20 sec, then go again. Switch legs that you start with on the next set to keep things even.
Shoulders	Dumbbell Shoulder Press	1	10-x-x	A good technique is to sit backwards in the Preacher bench so that the pad hits you in the mid-back rather than using the shoulder press bench with the vertical back. You'll get more back support this way.
Hamstrings	Leg Curls or Stiff-Legged Deadlifts	1	10-x-x	Leg Curls are a good option here as we can save the Stiff-Legged Deadlifts for the lower-rep day, which they're more suited to.
Traps	Barbell or Dumbbell Shrugs	1	10-x-x	With barbell shrugs, grip assistance is a good idea so that you work the traps without grip becoming an issue.
	Core Combo	4	-	2 sets of abs - 1 set of lower back - 1 set rotator cuff

General Comments:

- You will be using the Rest-Pause Training style today. Start with 10 reps on your first set, then rest 20 seconds, then go back to the same exercise and get as many more reps as you can (this might be about 3 to 5 reps - this is the "x" in the Reps section), rest 20 seconds, then get as many more reps as you can (maybe 2 to 3 reps).

- One time through these three sections is ONE rest-pause set.

- Take 90 seconds rest between rest-pause sets here.

Your Written Notes:

_____

_____

Mad Scientist Muscle - Day 10 - Rest

Body part	Exercise	Sets	Reps	Notes
None				

Cardiovascular Training	
Activity	Comments

General Comments:

Your Written Notes:

_____

_____

_____

_____

Nick Nilsson

Mad Scientist Muscle - Day 11 - Rest-Pause Training

Body part	Exercise	Rounds	Reps	Notes
Chest	Incline/Decline Barbell Bench Press or Dumbbell Bench Press	3	5-x-x	Dumbbell bench press can be done on the Swiss ball here. If you decide to go with barbell presses, use either Incline or Decline, to switch it up from the flat bench.
Back	Weighted Chin-Ups, Pulldowns, Barbell Rows, One-Arm Dumbbell Rows or Deadlifts	3	5-x-x	If you did Deadlifts on Day 1, go with one of the other exercises here, and go with Squats tomorrow.
Biceps	Barbell, Preacher or Dumbbell Curls	1	5-x-x	Any of these exercises is fine here. You're just doing one rest-pause set so make it count.
Calves	Standing, Donkey or Seated Calf Raises	1	5-x-x	When doing calf raises, hold the stretch at the bottom and the contraction at the top for a few seconds each, to maxmize the tension on the calves.
	Core Combo	4	-	2 sets of abs - 1 set of lower back - 1 set rotator cuff

General Comments:

- You will be using the Rest-Pause Training style today. Start with 5 reps on your first set, then rest 20 seconds, then go back to the same exercise and get as many more reps as you can (this might be about 2-3 reps - this is the "x" in the Reps section), rest 20 seconds, then get as many more reps as you can (maybe 1 or 2 reps).
- One time through these three sections is ONE rest-pause set.
- Take 90 seconds rest between rest-pause sets here.

Your Written Notes:

_____

_____

_____

_____

Mad Scientist Muscle - Day 12 - Rest-Pause Training

Body part	Exercise	Rounds	Reps	Notes
Shoulders	Barbell Hang Clean and Press or Military Press	1	5-x-x	The Hang Clean and Press is a good one here. It's better suited to lower-rep, explosive training.
Triceps	Decline Close Grip Bench Press or Weighted Dips	1	5-x-x	Decline Close Grip Press is great for loading the triceps with heavy weight. You can also use flat Close Grip Press, if you prefer.
Thighs	Squats or Leg Press	2	5-x-x	The preferred exercise here is the Squat. Leg Press will work if you're not physically able to squat, but you'll get more out of the Barbell Squat as an overall mass-builder.
Hamstrings	Stiff-Legged Deadlifts or Leg Curls	1	5-x-x	Stiff-Legged Deadlifts are the preferred option here. They're well-suited to lower-rep, heavier training.
Traps	Barbell or Dumbbell Shrugs	1	5-x-x	With barbell shrugs, grip assistance is a good idea so that you work the traps without grip becoming an issue.
	Core Combo	4	-	2 sets of abs - 1 set of lower back - 1 set rotator cuff

General Comments:

- You will be using the Rest-Pause Training style today. Start with 5 reps on your first set, then rest 20 seconds, then go back to the same exercise and get as many more reps as you can (this might be about 2-3 reps - this is the "x" in the Reps section), rest 20 seconds, then get as many more reps as you can (maybe 1 or 2 reps).

- One time through these three sections is ONE rest-pause set.

- Take 90 seconds rest between rest-pause sets here.

Your Written Notes:

_____

_____

_____

_____

Nick Nilsson

Mad Scientist Muscle - Day 13 & 14 - Rest

Body part	Exercise	Sets	Reps	Notes
None				

Cardiovascular Training	
Activity	**Comments**
Aerobic Interval Training	This is an OPTIONAL cardio training session done on Day 13 <u>ONLY.</u> Go for 15 to 20 minutes using any of the work to rest intervals listed on the Aerobic Interval Training page, e.g. 2 minutes work to 30 seconds rest intervals. The idea here is not to push yourself hard but to just maintain cardio capacity.

General Comments:

- The cardio training for this day is optional. If you find that doing cardio slows down muscle growth, you can opt not to do it.

- From a nutritional standpoint, treat your cardio session as a regular training session and have a post-workout meal and supplementation.

Your Written Notes:

_____

_____

_____

_____

Mad Scientist Muscle - Day 15 - Rest-Pause Training

Body part	Exercise	Rounds	Reps	Notes
Back	Deadlifts, Chin-Ups, Barbell Rows or One-Arm Dumbbell Rows	3	10-x-x	Deadlifts are the preferred exercise here since they involve the most muscle mass.
Chest	Barbell Bench Press or Dumbbell Bench Press	3	10-x-x	When doing barbell bench, be sure you don't flare your elbows out wide to the side at the bottom. Keep them tucked in towards your body a bit to save your shoulders.
Biceps	Barbell, Preacher or Dumbbell Curls	2	10-x-x	Any of these exercises is fine here. You're just doing one rest-pause set so make it count.
Calves	Standing, Donkey or Seated Calf Raises	2	10-x-x	When doing calf raises, hold the stretch at the bottom and the contraction at the top for a few seconds each, to maxmize the tension on the calves.
	Core Combo	4	-	2 sets of abs - 1 set of lower back - 1 set rotator cuf

General Comments:

- You will be using the Rest-Pause Training style today. Start with 10 reps on your first set, then rest 20 seconds, then go back to the same exercise and get as many more reps as you can (this might be about 3 to 5 reps - this is the "x" in the Reps section), rest 20 seconds, then get as many more reps as you can (maybe 2 to 3 reps).

- One time through these three sections is ONE rest-pause set.

- Take 1 minute rest between rest-pause sets here.

Your Written Notes:

_____

_____

_____

_____

Mad Scientist Muscle - Day 16 - Rest-Pause Training

Body part	Exercise	Rounds	Reps	Notes
Triceps	Weighted Dips, Close Grip Bench Press or Lying Tricep Extensions	2	10-x-x	Dips are the preferred exercise here. Keep your elbows in close to your body and keep your torso upright in order to focus the stress on the triceps over the chest.
Thighs	Front Squats or Dumbbell Split Squats	3	10-x-x	The preferred exercise here is the Front Squat. If you use DB Split Squats, do 10 reps on one leg, then 10 reps on the other, then take 20 sec, then go again. Switch legs that you start with on the next set to keep things even.
Shoulders	Dumbbell Shoulder Press	2	10-x-x	A good technique is to sit backwards in the Preacher bench so that the pad hits you in the mid-back rather than using the shoulder press bench with the vertical back. You'll get more back support this way.
Hamstrings	Leg Curls or Stiff-Legged Deadlifts	2	10-x-x	Leg Curls are a good option here as we can save the Stiff-Legged Deadlifts for the lower-rep day, which they're more suited to.
Traps	Barbell or Dumbbell Shrugs	1	10-x-x	With barbell shrugs, grip assistance is a good idea so that you work the traps without grip becoming an issue.
	Core Combo	4	-	2 sets of abs - 1 set of lower back - 1 set rotator cuff

General Comments:

- You will be using the Rest-Pause Training style today. Start with 10 reps on your first set, then rest 20 seconds, then go back to the same exercise and get as many more reps as you can (this might be about 3 to 5 reps - this is the "x" in the Reps section), rest 20 seconds, then get as many more reps as you can (maybe 2 to 3 reps).

- One time through these three sections is ONE rest-pause set.

- Take 1 minute rest between rest-pause sets here.

Your Written Notes:

_____

_____

Mad Scientist Muscle - Day 17 - Rest

Body part	Exercise	Sets	Reps	Notes
None				

Cardiovascular Training	
Activity	Comments

General Comments:

Your Written Notes:

_____

_____

_____

_____

Mad Scientist Muscle - Day 18 - Rest-Pause Training

Body part	Exercise	Rounds	Reps	Notes
Chest	Incline/Decline Barbell Bench Press or Dumbbell Bench Press	3	5-x-x	Dumbbell bench press can be done on the Swiss ball here. If you decide to go with barbell presses, use either Incline or Decline, to switch it up from the flat bench.
Back	Weighted Chin-Ups, Pulldowns, Barbell Rows, One-Arm Dumbbell Rows or Deadlifts	3	5-x-x	If you did Deadlifts on Day 1, go with one of the other exercises here, and go with Squats tomorrow.
Biceps	Barbell, Preacher or Dumbbell Curls	2	5-x-x	Any of these exercises is fine here. You're just doing one rest-pause set so make it count.
Calves	Standing, Donkey or Seated Calf Raises	2	5-x-x	When doing calf raises, hold the stretch at the bottom and the contraction at the top for a few seconds each, to maxmize the tension on the calves.
	Core Combo	4	-	2 sets of abs - 1 set of lower back - 1 set rotator cuff

General Comments:

- You will be using the Rest-Pause Training style today. Start with 5 reps on your first set, then rest 20 seconds, then go back to the same exercise and get as many more reps as you can (this might be about 2-3 reps - this is the "x" in the Reps section), rest 20 seconds, then get as many more reps as you can (maybe 1 or 2 reps).
- One time through these three sections is ONE rest-pause set.
- Take 1 minute rest between rest-pause sets here.

Your Written Notes:

_____

_____

_____

_____

Mad Scientist Muscle - Day 19 - Rest-Pause Training

Body part	Exercise	Rounds	Reps	Notes
Shoulders	Barbell Hang Clean and Press or Military Press	1	5-x-x	The Hang Clean and Press is a good one here. It's better suited to lower-rep, explosive training.
Triceps	Decline Close Grip Bench Press or Weighted Dips	1	5-x-x	Decline Close Grip Press is great for loading the triceps with heavy weight. You can also use flat Close Grip Press, if you prefer.
Thighs	Squats or Leg Press	2	5-x-x	The preferred exercise here is the Squat. Leg Press will work if you're not physically able to squat, but you'll get more out of the Barbell Squat as an overall mass-builder.
Hamstrings	Stiff-Legged Deadlifts or Leg Curls	1	5-x-x	Stiff-Legged Deadlifts are the preferred option here. They're well-suited to lower-rep, heavier training.
Traps	Barbell or Dumbbell Shrugss	1	5-x-x	With barbell shrugs, grip assistance is a good idea so that you work the traps without grip becoming an issue.
	Core Combo	4	-	2 sets of abs - 1 set of lower back - 1 set rotator cuff

General Comments:

- You will be using the Rest-Pause Training style today. Start with 5 reps on your first set, then rest 20 seconds, then go back to the same exercise and get as many more reps as you can (this might be about 2-3 reps - this is the "x" in the Reps section), rest 20 seconds, then get as many more reps as you can (maybe 1 or 2 reps).

- One time through these three sections is ONE rest-pause set.

- Take 1 minute rest between rest-pause sets here.

Your Written Notes:

_____

_____

Mad Scientist Muscle - Day 20 & 21 - Rest

Body part	Exercise	Sets	Reps	Notes
None				

Cardiovascular Training	
Activity	**Comments**
Aerobic Interval Training	This is an OPTIONAL cardio training session done on Day 20 <u>ONLY</u>. Go for 15 to 20 minutes using any of the work to rest intervals listed on the Aerobic Interval Training page, e.g. 2 minutes work to 30 seconds rest intervals. The idea here is not to push yourself hard but to just maintain cardio capacity.

General Comments:

- The cardio training for this day is optional. If you find that doing cardio slows down muscle growth, you can opt not to do it.
- From a nutritional standpoint, treat your cardio session as a regular training session and have a post-workout meal and supplementation.

Your Written Notes:

_____

_____

_____

_____

Mad Scientist Muscle - Day 1 - Triple Add Sets

Body part	Exercise	Rounds	Reps	Notes
Chest	Flat Barbell Bench Press or Dumbbell Press	2	20-30+ 6-8 1-3	Dumbbells are easier to work with on this training but barbells are good, too...it just takes time to add plates between sets.
Back	Close Grip or Wide Grip Pulldowns, Seated Cable Rows or Deadlifts	2	20-30+ 6-8 1-3	Selectorized machines are very useful for this type of training. T-Bar rows will also work well for this. You can also do with deadlifts - it'll just take a bit of time to add weight to the bar.
Biceps	Dumbbell Curls, Cable Curls or Barbell Curls	2	20-30+ 6-8 1-3	Dumbbell curls are the best choice for this style of training. When doing the light sets, start with both arms at the same time then move to single-arm alternating as you get tired. The next two parts should be done alternating arms.
Calves	Pushdowns, Dips, Close Grip Bench Press (flat or decline)	2	20-30+ 6-8 1-3	Pushdowns work well for this because of the weight stack. Dips can also be effective because you can hold dumbbells between your feet to add weight very quickly and easily to the movement. You'll need to be able to do 20+ bodyweight dips to use it, though.
	Core Combo	4	-	2 sets of abs - 1 set of lower back - 1 set rotator cuff

General Comments:

- Your first weight should allow around 20-30+ reps. Rest 10 seconds. Increase to a moderate weight and do 6-8 reps. Rest 10 seconds. Increase to a heavy weight and do 1-3 reps. This hits all the different muscle fibers in one shot.

- Dumbbell and selectorized cable exercises will be good choices for this but barbells can be very useful as well - just add the plates as quickly as you can and get right back to the exercise.

- Take 2 minutes rest between each set.

- You can switch up the exercises that you use the second week through on this style of training.

Your Written Notes:

_____

_____

Mad Scientist Muscle - Day 2 - Triple Add Sets

Body part	Exercise	Rounds	Sets/Reps	Notes
Thighs	Leg Press, Squats, Goblet Squats or DB Split Squats	2	20-30+ 6-8 1-3	The Leg Press doesn't require stabilization. Squats are also good - the only hitch is adding barbell plates on each set. Goblet squats - hold a db vertically in front you with your hands under the plates.
Shoulders	Dumbbell Shoulder Press or Military Press	2	20-30+ 6-8 1-3	When doing dumbbell presses, I recommend using the Preacher bench sitting with your back to the pad. It allows for better support and positioning in the exercise.
Hamstrings	Leg Curls or Stiff-Legged Deadlifts	2	20-30+ 6-8 1-3	Leg Curls are the better option here. SLDL's will be tough on the high-rep portion of the training. Definitely doable, though, if you don't have access to a leg curl machine.
Calves	Standing or Seated Calf Raises	1	20-30+ 6-8 1-3	In the high-rep portion, do the reps fast, without pausing. When you get to the medium and lower rep portions, that's when you should slow down and get the stretch and the contraction.
Traps	Barbell or Dumbbell Shrugs	1	20-30+ 6-8 1-3	Use a powerful, explosive movement for shrugs. Dumbbells are a good choice here.
	Core Combo	4	-	2 sets of abs - 1 set of lower back - 1 set rotator cuff

General Comments:

- Your first weight should allow around 20-30+ reps. Rest 10 seconds. Increase to a moderate weight and do 6-8 reps. Rest 10 seconds. Increase to a heavy weight and do 1-3 reps. This hits all the different muscle fibers in one shot.

- Dumbbell and cable exercises will be good choices for this - barbells can be very useful as well - just add the plates as quickly as you can.

- Take 2 minutes rest between each set.
- You can switch up the exercises that you use the second week through on this style of training.

Your Written Notes:

_____

_____

_____

_____

Mad Scientist Muscle - Day 4 - Low-Rep Strength Training

Body part	Exercise	Rounds	Reps	Notes
Chest	Flat Barbell Bench Press or Dumbbell Press	3	5-3-1	Don't let your elbows flare out as you lower the weight. Be sure to keep your shoulder blades tight in behind your back.
Back	Deadlifts, One Arm DB Rows or Weighted Chins	3	5-3-1	Don't let your lower back round over when performing deadlifts. If you did Deadlifts in the Triple Add Sets, don't use them here.
Biceps	Barbell Curls	3	5-3-1	Keep your knees slightly bent and keep your entire body tight. A loose body will lead to cheating reps.
Calves	Close Grip Bench Press (flat or decline) or Weighted Dips	3	5-3-1	Decline close grip bench will allow you to load more weight onto the triceps.
	Core Combo	4	-	2 sets of abs - 1 set of lower back - 1 set rotator cuff

General Comments:

- You'll be doing 3 sets for each body part...5 reps on the first set, 3 reps on the second set and 1 rep on the third set. Increase the weight on each set, unless you don't hit the target reps.
- Take 90 seconds to 2 minutes rest between each set.
- Don't push to failure on any sets. Always keep the do-or-die rep in you.
- You can switch up the exercises that you use the second week through on this style of training.

Your Written Notes:

_____

_____

_____

_____

Mad Scientist Muscle - Day 5 - Low-Rep Strength Training

Body part	Exercise	Rounds	Sets/Reps	Notes
Thighs	Barbell Squats, Front Squats or Leg Press	3	5-3-1	If you did Deadlifts the previous day, you can still do Barbell Squats here... you just might find your numbers are a bit lower. Front Squats are a good option here as well.
Shoulders	Seated Dumbbell Shoulder Presses, Miltary Press or Hang Clean and Press	3	5-3-1	Use strict form on these - don't overload the weight at the expense of good form and really feeling the shoulders perform the movement.
Hamstrings	Stiff-Legged Deadlifts or Good Mornings	3	5-3-1	SLDL'S are perfect here. If you're comfortable doing Good Mornings, these are also an excellent posterior chain exercise that hit the hamstrings well.
Calves	Standing, Donkey or Seated Calf Raises	3	5-3-1	Hold the top and bottom positions of the calf raise for at least 2 to 3 seconds to maximize the effect.
Traps	Barbell or Dumbbell Shrugs	3	5-3-1	Use a powerful, explosive movement for shrugs.
	Core Combo	4	-	2 sets of abs - 1 set of lower back - 1 set rotator cuff

General Comments:

- You'll be doing 3 sets for each body part...5 reps on the first set, 3 reps on the second set and 1 rep on the third set. Increase the weight on each set, unless you don't hit the target reps.

- Take 90 seconds to 2 minutes rest between each set.

- Don't push to failure on any sets. Always keep the do-or-die rep in you.

- You can switch up the exercises that you use the second week through on this style of training.

Your Written Notes:

_____

_____

_____

Mad Scientist Muscle

Mad Scientist Muscle - Day 6 and 7 - Rest

Body part	Exercise	Sets	Reps	Notes
None				

Cardiovascular Training	
Activity	**Comments**
Aerobic Interval Training	This is an OPTIONAL cardio training session done on Day 6 ONLY. Go for 15 to 20 minutes using any of the work to rest intervals listed on the Aerobic Interval Training page, e.g. 2 minutes work to 30 seconds rest intervals. The idea here is not to push yourself hard but to just maintain cardio capacity.

General Comments:

- The cardio training for this day is optional. If you find that doing cardio slows down muscle growth, you can opt not to do it.
- From a nutritional standpoint, treat your cardio session as a regular training session and have a post-workout meal and supplementation

Your Written Notes:

_____

_____

_____

_____

References

1. **Impact of acute exercise intensity on pulsatile growth hormone release in men.**

   J Appl Physiol. 1999 Aug;87(2):498-504. Pritzlaff CJ, Wideman L, Weltman JY, Abbott RD, Gutgesell ME, Hartman ML, Veldhuis JD, Weltman A.

2. **Hormonal responses of multiset versus single-set heavy-resistance exercise protocols.**

   Can J Appl Physiol. 1997 Jun;22(3):244-55. Gotshalk LA, Loebel CC, Nindl BC, Putukian M, Sebastianelli WJ, Newton RU, Hakkinen K, Kraemer WJ.

3. **Acute effects of high fat and high glucose meals on the growth hormone response to exercise.**

   J Clin Endocrinol Metab. 1993 Jun;76(6):1418-22. Cappon JP, Ipp E, Brasel JA, Cooper DM.

4. **Growth hormone responses during intermittent weight lifting exercise in men.**

   Eur J Appl Physiol Occup Physiol. 1984;53(1):31-4. Vanhelder WP, Radomski MW, Goode RC.

5. **Rapid carbohydrate loading after a short bout of near maximal-intensity exercise.**

   Med Sci Sports Exerc. 2002 Jun;34(6):980-6. Fairchild TJ, Fletcher S, Steele P, Goodman C, Dawson B, Fournier PA.

6. Timing Of Amino Acid-Carbohydrate Ingestion Alters Anabolic Response Of Muscle To Resistance Exercise.

American Journal Of Physiology & Endocrinology Metabolism, 281:E197-E206, 2001. Tipton KD, Rasmussen BB, Miller SL, et al.

7. A carbohydrate loading regimen improves high intensity, short duration exercise performance.

Int J Sport Nutr. 1995 Jun;5(2):110-6. Pizza FX, Flynn MG, Duscha BD, Holden J, Kubitz ER.

8. Adaptations to short-term high-fat diet persist during exercise despite high carbohydrate availability.

Med Sci Sports Exerc. 2002 Jan;34(1):83-91. Burke LM, Hawley JA, Angus DJ, Cox GR, Clark SA, Cummings NK, Desbrow B, Hargreaves M.

9. The effects of protein and amino acid supplementation on performance and training adaptations during ten weeks of resistance training.

J Strength Cond Res. 2006 Aug;20(3):643-53. Kerksick CM, Rasmussen CJ, Lancaster SL, Magu B, Smith P, Melton C, Greenwood M, Almada AL, Earnest CP, Kreider RB.

10. Effects of dietary leucine supplementation on exercise performance.

Eur J Appl Physiol. 2006 Aug;97(6):664-72. Epub 2005 Oct 29. Crowe MJ, Weatherson JN, Bowden BF.

11. Leucine supplementation and intensive training. Literature Review

Sports Med. 1999 Jun;27(6):347-58. Mero A.

12. Regional changes in capillary supply in skeletal muscle of high- intensity endurance-trained rats.

J Appl Physiol. 1996 Aug;81(2):619-26. Gute D, Fraga C, Laughlin MH, Amann JF.

13. Growth hormone stimulates the collagen synthesis in human tendon and skeletal muscle without affecting myofibrillar protein synthesis.

J Physiol. 2010 Jan 15;588(Pt 2):341-51. Epub 2009 Nov 23. Doessing S, Heinemeier KM, Holm L, Mackey AL, Schjerling P, Rennie M, Smith K, Reitelseder S, Kappelgaard AM, Rasmussen MH, Flyvbjerg A, Kjaer M.

14. From mechanical loading to collagen synthesis, structural changes and function in human tendon.

Scand J Med Sci Sports. 2009 Aug;19(4):500-10. Kjaer M, Langberg H, Heinemeier K, Bayer ML, Hansen M, Holm L, Doessing S, Kongsgaard M, Krogsgaard MR, Magnusson SP.

Suggested Reading

1. Dual Factor Training: How To Use Training Theory To Reach Your Physique & Performance Goals.

By Matt Reynolds

2. How to Benefit From Planned Overtraining

By Kelly Baggett

Index

Pure Physique

HOW TO MAXIMIZE FAT-LOSS- AND MUSCLULAR DEVELOPMENT

Pure Physique is for anyone who ever felt they should be getting more from their efforts in and out of the gym. This book will teach you how to put together an exercise and nutrition program that is truly tailor-fitted to meet your individual needs and goals. Unlike other books that provide fad diets and 'canned' workout routines, Pure Physique was designed with the individual in mind. With this book, you will finally be able obtain the leaner, more muscular body you've always wanted.

Unlike most books in the exercise and nutrition market, this book addresses how to account for differences in needs, goals, abilities, limitations, and preferences.

PURE PHYSIQUE

How to
MAXIMIZE
FAT-LOSS
and
MUSCULAR
DEVELOPMENT

Michael Lipowski

About the Author

Michael Lipowski is a certified fitness clinician and the President of the International Association of Resistance Trainers. He is a competitive natural Bodybuilder in the INBF, a consultant to other drug-free body builders, and was the personal trainer of the winner of the 2009 Men's Fitness Fit-to-Fat competition. Michael is a writer for Natural Bodybuilding & Fitness and has written for a number of other health and fitness publications worldwide.

ISBN-13/EAN:	9780972410274
Retail Price:	$14.95
Size:	6" x 9"
Page count:	224

Available on Amazon.com and Bookstores nationwide

"If you are like me and have been working out for years and wonder why you have stopped putting on muscle, then this book is for you. It will change the way you work out... It shed a whole new light on why people spend countless hours week in, week out, year after year in the gym lifting weights and not really changing their physique."

– TheHealthyBoy.com

MUSCLE EXPLOSION
28 DAYS TO MAXIMUM MASS

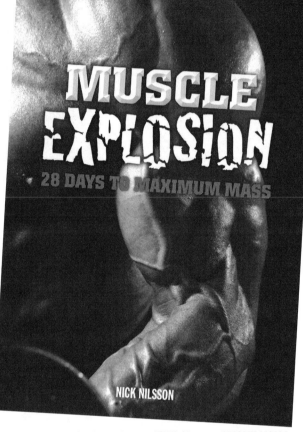

If you are part of the "conventional wisdom crowd," take a very deep breath… with Muscle Explosion you're going to:

- Reduce caloric intake to well below maintenance levels and eliminate protein completely (in very specific ways for very specific purposes)
- Aim to overtrain
- Train the same body part five days in a row
- Perform the same exercise five days in a row

Muscle Explosion literally turns conventional muscle-building wisdom inside-out and upside down. By practicing the groundbreaking training and eating strategies in this book, you will SHATTER your "genetic limitations" by literally changing your physiology, quickly setting the stage for EXPLOSIVE increases in muscle mass and strength.

Each cycle of this program lasts only 28 days and the workouts take less than an hour to complete. This book is for the intermediate to advanced trainer who is ready to DEMOLISH plateaus and achieve growth and strength increases previously thought unattainable.

ISBN-13:	9780972410298
Retail Price:	$14.95
Size:	7" x 10"
Page Count:	224

About the Author

Nick Nilsson, "The Mad Scientist" of the fitness world, is a renowned personal trainer, body builder, and professional fitness writer who has written for Men's Fitness, Reps Magazine, Muscle & Fitness and hundreds of fitness websites all over the internet. He is recognized throughout the fitness world as an innovator and pioneer of ground-breaking methods for building muscle and strength fast. His degree in physical education covers advanced biomechanics, physiology and kinesiology.

Available on Amazon.com and Bookstores nationwide

"Nick has developed the most effective training techniques that offer the greatest physiological gains in the shortest time possible." – *Exercise for Men Only* magazine March 2011